Come Home To Your Body

Workbook revised for Women Over 50

Connect Body, Mind and Spirit
for Anti-aging, Healing and Self-love

Pam Free

COME HOME TO YOUR BODY

PAM FREE

Disclaimer: The author and publisher of this book is not a medical professional. You must allow your own body wisdom to be your guide in doing any of the exercises.

Cover art by Pam Free

Healthy Over 50 Inc
www.healthyover50.com

COMING HOME TO MY BODY

As a child, I tumbled and twirled, danced, walked on my hands,
swung upside down from iron railings,
did headstands, handstands, cartwheels.
Dreamed of joining the circus, flying on a trapeze.
"Don't take any notice," said my sister, Diane,
"she can't help it, she's double-jointed."

Then came puberty, red blood flowing, strange and unexpected.
Keep my knees together, keep my feet on the floor,
grow up, act my age, behave myself,
walk like a lady, sit up straight,
everyone is looking at me, I'm not doing it right.
Shame! Shame! Shame!
I'll just leave my body.

I missed so many years of the rhythms of my body.
The ebbing and the flowing, the stretching and the growing,
all my systems circulating in their own mysterious patterns.
Muscles, glands, organs, blood and breath,
all pulsing and oozing, squeezing and leaping.
Magical transitions from desire into impulse into movement.
One thought creating a trillion interactions in the patterns of my cells,
leading to my arms going up or my feet going down.
Each time my hand reaches out for another
there occurs a miracle of so many dimensions,
energy and aura, muscle and bone, longing and yearning,
all translating into simple action.
How could I have been absent for so long
from my own true self?

No time now for regret.
Only time to pay attention.
To bring my awareness to the pleasure of being the Prodigal Daughter
returned to my own loving arms.
The exquisite sensations of skin, the languorous joy of muscles stretching,
the intensity of energy dancing.
Time to roll on the floor, make circular movements,
explore, rejoice, experience, feel.
Come home to my body.

Pam Free

COME HOME TO YOUR BODY

CONTENTS

INTRODUCTION

T his book grew out of my intensive work with women over the last thirty years. I have watched a huge shift in consciousness over those years, in myself and in my clients, as both the world of women and the external world have changed so rapidly. I have heard the voices of women from all walks of life calling for a way to correct the imbalance in their lives.

Women are ready to recognize and acknowledge their yearning to regain contact with their bodies from the inside. To live from within their body and heart wisdom. Body, mind, and Spirit, all must be connected and acknowledged in our daily lives for us to feel joy and inner peace, health and vitality. The current dominance of the mind over the body, and the ignoring of our spirituality, has left an empty space inside us for disease and disharmony to grow.

Now, moving into menopause and beyond, women still have the pivotal role in the family as nurturer and caregiver. Yet they also have a role in the redirection of the priorities on this planet before it is destroyed beyond recovery. We can't move into this role completely until we connect deeply to our bodies and our hearts, and to Earth and nature.

1

For many of us now our children are finally grown and leaving home, some leaving later than any previous generation. Some of us have accumulated a significant amount of possessions from all these years of work, while others are still struggling financially from losses due to divorce or sickness.

We all have our individual life dramas and special circumstances laying claim to our attention. But wherever women are gathered together, speaking from their hearts, I have heard a new willingness to stop and take stock of their lives in a meaningful way. We yearn for some sign of movement forward into the earned space of "Wise Woman," and dread instead the downward spiral into the dishonored role of "Old Woman."

We look at our health and our sense of well-being and we often find it lacking. Over the years of coping with too much work and too little time, the one part of our lives that could most easily be shoved aside was self-care, self-nurturing. We put everyone and everything ahead of our connection with ourselves. It was easier to stuff our feelings away with food or other addictions so we didn't feel our own inner pain.

Some women think they are in contact with their bodies because they take care of them as they would a fine car—they feed them right, exercise them regularly, get them checked over, and take pride in their accomplishments and appearance. But this is often done with a sense of separation, of ownership. The mind, the smart part, is taking care of the body, the dumb part, that they need to carry them around. Whether they do it from vanity or good sense, the caring does not come from within the body's own wisdom.

From the outside, from the mind and the will, we impose diets and exercise that are foreign to the body's true needs. This is from the belief that I *own* my body. This is treating our bodies as objects or possessions. The unspoken agreement is: I will take good care of it and it will work for me. When that agreement is violated by accident or illness, we are often outraged and deeply frightened. From my weight vest for Osteoporosis site I speak with many women who have just received a diagnosis of Osteopenia or Osteoporosis and they can't believe it. It brings up a huge fear reaction; partly because of drug companies fear-mongering and partly because it may be the first time they have looked aging in the eye. Aging is what happens to their mothers, not them!

So our first signs of aging are disillusioning. We can't trade our body in for a new model at the first dent or sign of shabbiness. Coming home to our body means to understand that we *are* our body, that body wisdom is far deeper and wiser than the intellectual mind, and that we need our body's connection to the larger Universe of which we are an essential part. That connection will deepen with age and then it will be easier to let go of the mainstream ideas about beauty and looking right.

The universal gift of this time is to become aware of the dance of energy running through our bodies in every moment. Our bodies are actually the densest part of this energy, but we extend out far beyond the body. When we are asleep to the ebbs and flows of our own energy fields, we have little regard for the rhythms of our lives. We allow the dragon of time to rush us through our days on the hurry-up!

We are often equally out of touch with our kinesthetic senses—the sense of pleasure and comfort we get from touch. Most people in this society don't get touched enough. Women can get back in touch with sensory pleasure from within their own bodies so they can feel the flow of life from a centered place in their own belly. We can discover how to touch *ourselves* so that self-loving, creative, sensual energy flows unblocked within us.

This book can teach you how to be awake to the first sign of stress or discomfort so that changes can be made before disease becomes a reality in your life. Dis-ease is exactly what it says, lack of comfort in your body/mind. Many women I meet are so far out of touch with themselves that they no longer have any clear idea of what comfort or pleasure is, except in terms of the addictions that give us pleasure by numbing us to our discomfort.

When we are connected to our bodies we can experience joy in any moment; a windy day on the beach, a smile from a stranger, clearing our space, dancing through the house........the list is endless. Every movement becomes an exploration.

I invite you to wake up to the realization that our lives are out of balance, that peace of mind, comfort in the body, and connection with our own Spirit are not found outside ourselves. Let's look *inside* in ways that are natural to the feminine and find integration and peace.

4

1

HOW TO USE THIS BOOK

I SET THE INTENTION TO DO THE WORK OF CHANGE

For years I was unconsciously searching for the perfect female role model. Every time I read about mentors and role models I wanted one of my own. Someone who would lead me forward on my life path, show me the way, teach me the steps, and be my loving guide. Like many women of my generation, mine was a solitary path of growth. I felt alone and different much of the time, so I kept my antennae out for potential guides wherever I went. I think I wanted to grow up into one of those older women who do yoga and wear white and have long silver hair and are very spiritual.

Finally I realized that is not who I am. First of all white doesn't suit me, I love color! So I created a clear picture of that ideal woman I wanted to become, made up of all of the qualities I admire and wasn't acknowledging I already had. We will all have a different ideal image that completely reflects our own inner feminine.

So here is the vision I have to grow into:

- FuturePam is a powerful woman adding value to the world, she radiates love from Source most of the time and has a deep inner calm.

- She can act very decisively to create and reach her desires.

- She takes life's events in stride, responding with a sense of humor to all the blocks in her path, maybe after a tantrum or two.

- She can reach out to others and to life with love and passion, and also honor her own need to have time alone and time in nature.

- She makes choices from her own inner wisdom and creativity, and not from the tugging and pulling of others needs or the needs of her own inner child.

- Her body is strong, healthy, and flexible and has visible muscles and vitality.

I consider myself a work of art in progress. Sometimes I find I am sprinting along my path without a moment's hesitation, and other times I wander far afield, feeling lost and small and alone. But I couldn't move forward at all without my connection with my own body wisdom that has become my true guide. It is only because I know how to come home to my body, blending body, mind, and Spirit in harmony, that I can even dream of moving fully into FuturePam.

Take some time to create your own unique Futureself and see how much closer to her you feel after you have done all the work in the book.

What does it mean to *come home to your body?*

Remember a bad day you had recently when you hit the ground running and never did catch up. Everything you did was done in haste and didn't work out as you would have wished. You were crabby and tense, or you played out the martyr or victim role. That was a day run by your mind or negative emotions. You probably didn't check in with your body at all until some part of it hurt. It is likely that you were in some pain by the end of the day because no one was home taking care of your body. These are the days when accidents happen. We don't cut ourselves, fall down, or walk into fixed objects on days when we are centered in our bodies. We also don't destroy our relationships with hasty words.

Now remember a good day. It probably involved a slower pace or a sense of connectedness in your belly. You were moving from your center and you had time to laugh or talk with someone you love, or touch and be touched. Your heart was open and you felt more like reaching out to others. You could use your senses for pleasure, looking at people and finding them beautiful, smelling fresh air or hearing musical sounds, tasting rich and subtle flavors. All the necessary things got done effortlessly and you chose to be at peace with what didn't get done. You weren't tormented by impossible lists and perfectionist standards. This was a day of being more at home in your body. It could be called living from a heart-centered place.

We often can't change the external events in our lives. We have only limited power over others. People in your life will be the way they are and will do what is right for them. What we *can* change is our reaction to people and events, and we can bring the awareness of being centered in our body into even our craziest days.

That is what I hope you can teach yourself as you work through this book. I am sure you have heard a zillion times that the secret to happiness is to be in the NOW moment. Stop having and doing, and become a human *being*. What I have found with many of the women I have worked with over the years is that they don't have any idea how to go about the process of *being*, so they have no choice.

By using the simple tools in this book, you will eventually learn to use your body comfort as a constant guide in your life. You will be clear immediately when you have lost touch with your body, just as you would notice it right now if you stopped breathing or if your heart stopped beating.

So stop reading and *actually do* the exercises described in the text. Stretch your body/mind a little, make a leap and embody this new learning.

When I tell you a story, stop and look in your own memory bank. My stories are in the book in order to evoke your own stories, your own life experiences.

Use a notebook to record your thoughts, feelings, and experiences as you move through the book. I always think I will remember later but my journal is a better record.

Reading about concepts and ideas can evoke some productive inner dialog, but when you feel an experience in your own body/mind, then the new learning is yours forever. I was just given a quote I love from Benjamin Franklin,

"Tell me and I forget, teach me and I may remember, involve me and I learn."

My Own Journey

I want to begin by telling you a part of my own journey so you can see the path that has led to the writing of this book. During the seventies I was a supermom with a business of my own. I had six employees, I had an organic garden, I kept bees and chickens, and I remodeled the house in my spare time. I was a crazy type A woman with big dreams.

I worked all the time and I had ideas for more work streaming through my brain constantly. I was a successful, creative dynamo and didn't even realize how completely out of balance I was. My personal relationships were a disaster because I didn't understand why everyone didn't want to work as hard as I did. I was driven.

Someone I respected told me I needed to take a yoga class. I loved it passionately and the practice changed my life. Yoga started me on the path toward wholeness. Then I gradually came to realize that the underlying belief of this early form of yoga was that the spiritual life was all-important and the body was just a temple to house the soul. There was a denial of the vitality of the emotions and the power of the creative force of sexuality.

I started studying psychology and moved on to transformational psychology and energy work. Once again I loved it. It made such sense. I learned about the energy fields of the body; how to heal with energy, how to feel the energy fields of others. I was fascinated. Mystics say we all have a divine spark of unrest within us that drives us on to be the best we can be. I completely believe that. Never underestimate the power of this divine discontent within you. If you listen to this force it will lead you on, step by step, on the path of your growth.

Next I learned various forms of bodywork—Trager and massage. I wanted to be a healer and heal with my hands. I had been healing with energy for some time, but for many people this kind of healing was too esoteric and unstructured, even unbelievable. They could not *feel* the energy flow in their bodies.

At that time, the tools of bodywork and massage were understandable to more people. I felt I was getting closer to my goal. The problem this time was that people would come to me from their crazy lives, lie down on the table, and let me fix them. They got up feeling wonderful and went right back into their crazy lives. Since they didn't participate in any way in their own healing, they didn't stay fixed. The next week they were back again. I began to feel like a medic on the battlefield. Suddenly that story about giving a hungry woman a fish and she is fed for a day, but teach her how to fish and you have fed her for a lifetime, started to make really good sense to me.

I took some time out while I consumed everything I could find about every kind of alternative healing. Then I discovered the Feldenkrais Method. Named after the Israeli scientist who developed it, it is a method of teaching the brain by moving the body. By making very small and sometimes unusual movements, we can release blocks and pain in the body and learn new, more useful ways of interacting with our environment. The key is awareness. When you know what you are doing, you can do what you want, until then you are a puppet.

The work is about learning new choices, and it demands the interaction of the practitioner, as teacher, and the student. The Feldenkrais student has a completely different responsibility than the client of a healer. This student knows she is going to have to do the major part of the work of change. To me this was a big step in the right direction. I joined a training group and over a four-year period rolled around on the floor for hours making odd and wonderful movements. I connected with my body in the way I had been seeking for years. It was magical.

Feldenkrais had a very scientific mind. He thought energy work was New Age and therefore highly suspect, but since I already had that knowledge in my repertoire, this was the final link. I was home. Gradually, in my practice of

11

teaching rather than healing, I discovered and clarified my life purpose. I realized that the keys to my growth have been to listen to my inner wisdom and to trust my body, being willing to be present with it. When I am in this space I am completely aligned on my life path.

When I got very sick with chronic fatigue, candida and various other diseases, ending with diabetes 1 and Hashimotos thyroiditis, I never lost my ability to be comfortable in my body. I didn't have the energy I was used to but I didn't have pain or discomfort. It turned out after many years of searching that it was probably a mold reaction to a new living space that dropped me in my tracks. But I see it as a blessing. My whole life was turned around and I had time to go within and rediscover the essential me.

My mission is to teach other women how to contact *their* inner wisdom and connect with *their* bodies in a profound and lasting way, so that they can each find their own particular life path. We are all so miraculously unique and we each have our own life purpose, and yet we can all use the same simple tools of self-awareness to guide us. We are all headed in the same direction, toward the union of body, mind, and Spirit and to the awakening of the heart. The world needs us to do this work now so we can contribute to its transformation.

To begin at the beginning, I want to guide you step by step into being in the NOW moment. In this moment, what counts is being at home in your body, content and feeling connected with the rest of the Universe. You may have a chronic condition of dis-ease, such as arthritis, manifesting in your body, but that does not automatically prevent you from experiencing contentment. We all know people who are suffering from terrible physical ailments who are totally open and heart-centered, while others with the very same problem are acting out of the victim pattern. It doesn't matter what our particular life drama is about. It is possible to be in a state of inner peace and connection with both our body and our Spirit.

When I speak of Spirit I am speaking of the life force that runs through us but is much bigger than us, that connects us to the mystery of Source and to the larger dimensions of life. When we open to the part of us that is Spirit, we can see our life lessons more clearly and move out of the "Why me?" space into a larger perspective.

I was hesitant to mention the word Spirit in my work for many years. For some people it has a religious connotation and they immediately back away. Gradually I found that if I don't anchor my teaching and my healing to the larger dimension of who we are and what we are doing in *this* body at *this* time, the lessons don't stay learned. Our daily dramas are such a small, though compelling, part of who we are. The deeper parts of us, our Inner Wisdom and our Higher Self, are always waiting patiently for us to remember that.

Workbook Suggestions

Here are my recommendations for how to get the most out of this book. This is a WORKbook, so if you skip the exercises, it won't work for you. I have a friend who buys all the "right" books but never makes time to read them or do the work involved. We joke that she has the most evolved bookshelf on this planet.

Get a notebook and write down all that you notice as you work your way through the book. Writing is an interesting thing; some people love it and some people hate it. Anything we learned to do in school seems to evoke automatic resistance in some of us. This writing is for you alone. Don't bother with grammar or spelling or punctuation. Just put your pen to the paper and let your words spill out as if you were talking to yourself. If you get stuck, write the words "I am" or "I feel" and see what follows. You don't have to do it any certain way. Just write!

When I go over and over in my head about a problem, I never seem to be able to resolve it. The very act of writing it down always brings me more clarity. Also, my insights are right there in black and white if I get pulled into the same pattern again. It is amazing how repetitive our life dramas are and we often don't realize it until we write them down. In some sense, I always find that writing clears my slate and lets me start again, fresh and new and open.

Complete the chapters in order, one a week if possible. If you need more time then take it, but not so long that you lose momentum. If you are a person who learns slowly, then do one chapter a month or start a new chapter on each New Moon. By having a planned time period, you avoid drifting away from your purpose. If you hate or resist any particular chapter, notice that reaction. It's always very interesting to note what we resist; often it is the very thing we need to do the most, but give yourself permission to skip

14

it and take what you need. You may choose to come back to it later. If you were my client, I would tailor the experience just for you. So you can do that for yourself.

We all have different ways that are comfortable for us to learn new skills. I have tried to incorporate many choices. If you are a predominantly aural person, put some of the exercises on tape and listen to them. My chief bias is that the best way for anyone to learn is by personal experience. Sometimes we can remember experiences we have already had and look at them in a new way.

Each chapter begins with an affirmation. Write it out, big and in color, and stick it on your bathroom mirror and refrigerator door. Allow it to dance around in the back of your mind every day and say it before you go to sleep. Affirmations are a great way to utilize the enormous power of the mind. I don't ever intend to belittle that power when I push for more equality for body and Spirit.

If you could inspire a group of three or four women to work with you and meet once a week to share, it would be enormously helpful. We are all different and we are all alike. A support group can clarify things for you and save you time and pain by seeing things from a different perspective. Ask around but don't over-persuade. People who are pushed into it won't go the distance, and that could affect your determination. Women really supporting women in their growth is one of the most wonderful experiences we can share.

Moving into the world of business has caused many women to become competitive, but that is not our true nature. We are cooperative beings and we have been isolated for far too long. I have facilitated several groups of women of various kinds and I am always amazed at how much we all learn from each others experience. We don't have to reinvent the wheel. By resonating with another woman's experience we can see our own life stories in a new way. The love and support and honest feedback I got from my groups accelerated my growth and deeply enriched my life. I am enormously grateful for them.

Make a commitment to yourself to work through the whole book no matter what comes up in your life to interfere. The tools are designed to be done mostly during your normal life. They won't take an enormous amount of extra time from your schedule. On the few occasions when they do, you are worth it.

Be curious. Curiosity is vital to an interesting life. Remember how babies are endlessly curious. They play with their fingers and toes for hours. They try new things a trillion times before settling on the best way for them. If we had all given up at the third or fourth try, we would still be lying on our backs like beached turtles. You now become the object of your own curiosity. YOU are fascinating. How do you act? How do you move? What makes you feel good or bad? What reaction does a certain external event have on your physical body?

This isn't a scientific method. We will never get consensus and absolutely nothing is repeatable in exactly the same way. We are all unique at each unique moment in time. That alone is such a miracle. Learn to *trust* your own experiences. Don't take my word for anything. Don't give up too soon, and don't close your mind to new possibilities.

I never use statistics or footnotes because I don't believe in them. Statistics and studies can be quoted to prove anything, and also the opposite. There are plenty of books that are full of amazing statistics and studies about the body/mind connection, but for now I want you to have your own direct experience of each lesson. Remember that when you feel something in your own body, it is yours forever.

You will probably find that some chapters remind you of things you have done in the past or have heard a hundred times before, while some ideas may be completely new to you. See if you can move to "beginner's mind" with each exercise and do it as if it were the first time you have ever seen it. There is always a way to deepen our experience if we don't assume we already know all there is to know about a subject. Rather than thinking of the lessons of life as a ladder on which the tests become progressively harder as we move up, try to think of them as unfolding in layers, like the layers of an onion or the petals of a lotus, to reveal a new richness at each depth.

I have tried to keep both the information and the lessons as simple and direct as possible. Watching women among men, I am always struck by the sophistication of our language and the intellectual discussion of concepts and ideas, often with the swirling undercurrent of competition for attention. In groups of women, in a non-business setting, the language becomes simpler and more honest, sharing from the heart and from our emotions. We may cry, but we always laugh a lot. We love to tell our stories, the small vignettes of our lives that reveal us completely. It is this level I am trying to evoke in you. I ask simple questions so that you can look inside and rediscover your own history, your own mythology.

What this can do is change your life from the inside, as you live from a more integrated place. When your body, mind, and Spirit are in alignment, you have access to all the answers you need about healing the particular pains and lacks in your life. Your own body wisdom knows what you need to do to be happy and at peace with the world. We just can't hear the message over the constant chatter in our heads and in our lives.

One of my clients, Lynn, said that as she watched her mother in her eighties become more and more fragile, she was deeply afraid that she was following along on the same downward path. For her, this was a wake-up call. She woke up to her disconnection from her body. After doing the lessons in this book, and some other Feldenkrais work, she had renewed hope in her own ability to create a healthy future. We have enough ninety-year-old women as role models who are bursting with energy and health and still enjoying life to know that we have that choice, if we commit to taking care of our body/minds from this moment forward.

Moving into this chapter:

Get a notebook.

Set your intention to do the work necessary to change your life.

Set up a reward system, preferably non-addictive, for doing each chapter.

Find companions for the journey if you can.

Stay curious.

COME HOME TO YOUR BODY

2

TOOLS OF AWARENESS

WITH AWARENESS I AM PRESENT IN EACH MOMENT

The first lesson will work on awakening your self-awareness. In the normal sequence of learning, once an action or behavior is learned, it becomes more automatic and requires less attention. In this way, most actions and thoughts in our daily lives become habitual and move outside of our conscious awareness. Our body sensations, in particular, sink below the threshold of our conscious mind. We have all had the experience of walking or driving somewhere, deep in thought, and arriving without really knowing how we got there. Another common experience is to walk past someone we know without seeing them. We seem to be on automatic pilot during much of our daily lives.

This unconscious repetition of our habitual patterns is often very useful to us. If we tried to become conscious of every repetitive act we do in just one day we would go crazy, but without awareness there is no possibility of change. What we are going to practice this week is a special kind of selective awareness.

For example, right now you are reading this book. Your attention is focused on the written words. Now add to your awareness the body sensations of sitting, but without changing your sitting posture in any way. It's almost impossible, isn't it? The act of noticing itself will subtly change anything.

Try again. Notice your breathing. Is it high in your chest or deep in your belly? Are you hunched over in any way so that you have difficulty taking a full breath? As you thought about it, did you straighten up?

Notice the place on your spine between your shoulder blades. Are you holding tension there? Notice your shoulders. Are they up around your ears? Did you change them if they were?

Were you able to read this passage and notice your body sensations at the same time? In general, women have the ability to utilize multiple awareness because this is a function of the right side of the brain. Most of us can easily prepare a meal, listen to a conversation, and keep one eye on children playing, all at the same time.

Refining your ability to tune into your body sensations while you continue with your normal life will probably be relatively easy for you. The *value* in learning to include these sensations in your awareness lies in your ability to prevent chronic pain from becoming part of your reality. *Chronic* means pain that is long-standing, recurs again and again, or is always there but in varying degrees. Pain is a message from our body, and becomes chronic only when the message has been ignored for too long. Most pain, from accidents on the job, to carpal tunnel syndrome, to migraines, can be prevented long before it occurs by staying in constant touch with the comfort level of your body. Pain *is NOT* a necessary part of the aging process.

The primary tool of awareness is the habit of noticing. It is almost instantaneous, almost effortless, and yet can relieve your body of many of the stresses and strains of your daily life. Women customarily carry their stress in their shoulders or their hips. When do *you* normally pay attention to the tension in your shoulders? Is it after you get home from work, or just before bed as you finally let go of the day? Or is it only when the sensation becomes very painful? We have so many claims on our attention that it seems the claim of our body sensation is most often ignored.

Many years ago I had a stressful job and a long drive home. About thirty minutes after I left work, still thinking about my day, I would drive through a tunnel. Perhaps because of the darkness of the tunnel, I would suddenly notice my shoulders up next to my ears and consciously let them down with a sigh of relief. I got in the habit of using

23

the tunnel as a signal to change from my working self to my evening self, leaving my job concerns behind and letting go of the tension in my shoulders.

The trick to noticing is the curiosity I mentioned earlier. If it just another thing to remember to do in your day, you will probably resist it. Try thinking of noticing as a positive, interesting way to use your mind when you would otherwise be worrying about your problems. Instead of rerunning, for the hundredth time, the argument you are having with the imaginary person in your head, watch what your body is doing. That is one of the main differences between humans and animals. A cat is prepared in an instant to fight or flee danger, and when the danger is past, she doesn't sit and agonize about it, she gets back to full relaxation. We have such big, advanced brains that we get to replay our worst moments again and again.

Imagine that human beings and their behavior are one of the most intriguing and entertaining puzzles in the world. Have you ever caught yourself behaving in some way (yelling or nagging or flirting, for instance) and wondered who on earth got inside you? It is fascinating to watch ourselves use our bodies to interact with each other.

Notice the changes in your body posture when someone you are attracted to, or want to impress, approaches you. Learning to consciously read body language, both our own and others, is so useful. We all read each other all the time on an intuitive level already, bringing that skill into conscious awareness will benefit you enormously. When you start noticing your own behaviors through your body movements, you will starton a voyage of discovery that can last your whole life long.

One large problem with developing the habit of noticing is our old habit of self-judgment. You are probably aware that we all have an inner critic, a part of our subconscious mind that we created as a child. It is usually our internalized parent, so it can operate as either a loving guide or, very often, a harsh detractor. Since many of our parents were pretty unconscious about child rearing, it is usually safe to assume that your inner critic is often too picky and downright rude for your peace of mind. In fact, the inner critic is probably one of the reasons we went unconscious in the first place! So be very sure that you don't use noticing for extra ammunition to criticize yourself. There is no right or wrong here; you can leave out judgment entirely. This is not another opportunity to make yourself feel bad.

Go back to the time before you judged yourself as right or wrong, as a failure or a success. That would be a very young age for most of us. Our inner critic is born very early and gathers enormous power. Notice your feelings and actions now with the joyful spirit of curiosity and exploration.

Here is a simple example of this technique: I can notice that I habitually sit with my whole spine leaning on one elbow as I work at my desk. I now have choices:

- I can continue as I am.

- I can move to a more balanced position so I don't increase the tension in my shoulders and spine.

25

- I can nag at myself for sitting so poorly. Most of us have the "sit up straight" voice of our parents and early teachers deeply embedded in our bodies and minds.

If I notice that I often nag myself, this is valuable information. The inner critic often nags away at you in the background of your thoughts, taking the shine off your self-esteem without your conscious attention. I may choose to change this pattern of automatic self-blame in order to make my life more comfortable. It *is* possible to put your inner critic on reduced duty, a kind of semi-retired status. The first step toward doing that is to notice it.

If I utilize the second choice of adjusting my sitting posture into balance, then I could prevent future misalignment and probable pain. If I decide to keep on sitting and leaning, I am now doing it consciously. Whatever choice I make, I am winning. Noticing—bringing some act or behavior into the light of conscious awareness—is a winning strategy.

Noticing Effort

The first thing I have my clients notice is the amount of extra effort they put into their daily tasks. Many of them have said that this awareness alone started a process of change that led to great transformation.

Cathy was completely unaware of the level of tension she always held in her body. Her movements were jerky and stiff. She wondered why her muscles were always in knots and also why no one seemed comfortable when she was around. She said she would love to be relaxed and peaceful but she wasn't that kind of person and never had been. She lived alone and didn't really trust people to like her, so she had a hard time making friends. She started noticing small things about the effort she made in her movements and she said, "It is almost as if I am fighting with myself, deep down inside, about every movement I make. I think people are watching me when they aren't. When I do everything more gently, with less effort, the world seems to shift into another focus. I see things differently." Before long she was able to move out of her mind, back inside her body, and her outer life did transform.

How much effort do you put into doing your daily repetitive tasks, all the things you do mindlessly every day?

- Notice how tightly you hold your comb or your toothbrush.

- How firmly do you clasp your fork while eating?

- How firmly or gently do you place something on the table or desk?

- How hard do your feet hit the ground?

- Do you frown or make faces as you think?

- Do you look serious whenever you are doing work?

- How firmly do you hold the telephone to your ear?

- How aggressive are your gestures?

- How loud is your voice?

- Are your movements jerky or smooth?

- Are you usually in a hurry?

Many of us wear out our joints with extra effort, in the same way that jogging on concrete will wear out your knee and hip joints faster than walking on grass. The joints in our hands, wrists, and shoulders especially show the effects of a lifetime of holding on too tight.

The amount of effort we use also gives us clues to our emotional state. When we are peaceful and loving, our movements will tend to be smoother and softer.

I always knew when my mother was upset by the way she brushed my hair. My parents never argued in front of us, but some days I wished I were bald and I thought I probably soon would be. My mother would tug and jerk and pull on my frizzy permed curls until I screamed. She laughed about it when she became a laid back Californian, but the other women she worked with used to say, "Just get Joan mad and she'll work like ten men." Since her life was often frustrating, the floors were always polished, the brass gleamed, and the windows shone. It was unexpressed anger translating into effort.

During the learning phase of acquiring a new skill, it is normal to use more effort and involve more muscles than we need. We have all seen people with their faces scrunched up, learning how to write or draw. It doesn't help, actually. While learning to ride a bicycle, you can probably remember the fear that kept many of your muscles tight and tense and made it much harder for you to learn. Gradually, with practice, we move into the area of competence and start to relax all the muscles not necessary for completing the task.

Most of us stop at the level of competence and never go any further. In the case of biking, our bike is a tool to get us where we need to go. There are some people, however, who will fall in love with biking and they will move beyond competence into the level of the lyrical, where they and their bike become one. You can find videos on youtube of teenagers riding their bikes on railings and walls. To watch their effortless movement is a joy. They are in the flow space.

Is there anything that you do so well that you become lyrical and flowing and forget effort?

While noticing effort, you may also make the discovery that you don't put enough effort into what you do. Most women work too hard for their own good (a historical pattern), but there is an opposite pattern of insecurity that some of us show the world. Then we are so tentative, so soft, so gentle, that we seem ineffective at everything we do. We whisper when we talk, ask permission for everything, and apologize constantly. If you think this applies to you, even in one or two of your life roles, you could practice turning up the effort bit by bit until you get the respect every woman deserves. None of us has to apologize for being present. We all have our own unique collection of skills and talents, and we have as much right to be here as anyone else.

Spend the first two days of this week noticing the amount of effort you use without trying to change it.

Notice also what frame of mind or emotion seems to accompany excessive effort.

The next two days, experiment with varying your effort and finding out the minimum amount it takes to complete a task efficiently.

Notice if decreasing the work involved in many of your daily routine tasks makes an appreciable difference in your life. For many of my clients, just this small change is the beginning of the wake-up process.

Sit comfortably at a desk or table and pick up an object like a plastic or metal cup. Holding it as tight as possible, bang it down on the table forcefully Allow your attention to travel through your body while you are doing this until you are clear which muscles are tight and involved in this action, and which are not.

Do you notice anything happening in your jaw or your face? How about your thighs and buttocks? Are you feeling any emotion?

Now gradually ease off the force and effort, repeating the same movement more softly and gently. What changes? Are fewer muscles involved?

Now put the cup down as silently as possible and notice if the tension returns when you are trying too hard to achieve gentleness. At what point does the softness turn into an *effort* to be soft?

In the same way, it takes more effort to shout or to whisper than it does to talk within a normal range.

Now think of the words *grace* and *ease* and pick up and put down the cup with those qualities in your awareness.

Did the quality of your movement change again? Isn't grace the very absence of effort, the smooth flow of natural movement? The ideal movement is one that uses all the muscles that need to be used for its accomplishment and no more.

Grimacing or scowling as we write, or tightening our shoulders as we think, is called "parasitic movement." It is unnecessary action.

Can you imagine the amount of energy you would have left over at the end of the day if you always moved with grace, involving all the necessary muscles and the necessary effort and no more?

Most of the women I have worked with do not believe themselves to be graceful. Maybe it is a skewed sample since most are seeking help with movement or pain, but even the professional dancers I know often have the same belief.

Feldenkrais said that in movement we can make the impossible possible, the possible effortless, and the effortless elegant. But you can't achieve elegance and grace from the outside—from the mind. Your awareness has to be *inside* the body, and then elegance is effortless.

Many of us checked out of our bodies when we hit the gawky, clumsy stage at puberty—when we were embarrassed about our growth and bewildered by our hormonal changes. We confused our appearance with our essence, and a pimple became a tragedy.

31

Start checking back into your body on a regular basis. Pick one small movement you do often, like picking up your coffee cup, and make it smoother and more flowing. It isn't so very difficult to make our small everyday movements graceful. Experiment. Don't make hard work of it. You could be the first woman to make drinking tea a lyrical experience.

Now begin to notice the times when you do movements "to the maximum," even though going halfway would be enough. This is slightly different than over-efforting.

Try this: Stand up and raise your left arm to the ceiling. Try hard; do it to the max. What did you learn?

Now raise your aim very slowly and feel *how* you do it. Which part of you starts the motion, then what muscles kick in? When does your shoulder get involved? What are your eyes doing? Are you making faces? What are your feet doing to participate?

Don't stretch as far as you could. Instead of being goal-oriented, be process-oriented. It's a whole different experience.

It is wonderful and productive to have goals, but if we can't be present during the process of reaching them, then we have bypassed most of our lives.

After all, when you achieve a goal, what happens? You usually start out immediately toward another one. You may as well enjoy the journey.

Our culture encourages the habit of trying hard and doing everything to the maximum—it's part of our socialization.

Do your best!

Strive for perfection!

If at first you don't succeed, try, try try again!

This frantic striving can wear us out before our time because it doesn't take into account the ebbs and flows of life. Doing dishes isn't the same as doing microsurgery. Sometimes we can just settle back and coast. We can get by on less effort and stop wearing ourselves out with such high expectations. Then when it comes to the goals or tasks we care about deeply, we can use the extra energy we have to do our very best.

I've already admitted that I used to be a compulsive workaholic, and on some days I put out maximum effort at maximum speed for sixteen to eighteen hours. I would crawl into bed still feeling as if I had not accomplished enough. If only there were more hours in the day, I could have done it all.

Then a young woman came to work for me, and when I was obsessing about doing something perfectly she would say, "Pam, this is not brain surgery, is it? What will this matter in a hundred years?"

At first I was totally shocked. Her attitude was completely foreign to me, but gradually it started to make sense. Now she is a dear friend and our favorite saying is

33

"Life is too short." It's too short to spend in anything less than peace and happiness, with some passion thrown in. Don't wear yourself out on the small stuff. You wouldn't dream of cooking all your meals at 550 degrees. Back off on your own energy use; your body will last longer and you'll enjoy it more.

Moving into this chapter:

Practicing the art of noticing our body sensations and release any self-judgment.

Notice your effort, vary the level, and discover the amount needed to complete the task with ease.

34

3

BREATHING

MY BREATH CONNECTS ME WITH ALL LIFE

Everyone, without exception, who is reading this book is breathing. Breathing is absolutely vital to us and yet we are usually unconscious of it. It is the *quality* of our breath that determines how alive we are, how awake, how vivacious, even how interesting our life is. Learning to breathe correctly for each situation we are in is the fastest way to change our lives for the better. No matter what emotional or physical pain you are in right now breathing with awareness will help you to alleviate it. That is a pretty big claim for something so simple to learn, but it is absolutely true.

In my workshops, I often get resistance to breathwork; breathing is boring, I already know how to breathe, let's do something new and exciting.

Trust me, breathing is the road home to peace of mind, acceptance of your emotions, and the awakening of your body intuition. The exhalation of our breath is a metaphor for our life. If we can learn to exhale fully and completely, we will become attuned to the universal need to let go before we can truly begin again. Breathing is letting go, emptying out with the deep trust that the next breath will be there for us. Like the woman on top of a burning building, we have to let go completely before we can jump to safety. Isn't it amazing how many people choose to hold on to the old, to what is killing them, rather than to leap into the new?

In shallow chest breathing we hold on to our old breath and never fully exhale. Our blood doesn't get enough oxygen and every cell in our body, especially in the brain, is affected. Deep breathing can slow our brainwaves down to the alpha state. It is only then that we can access our deeper wisdom. Our normal beta brain rhythm is too active to give us time to pay attention to our quiet, powerful voice of inner knowing.

Why do we need to learn how to breathe? It is the same old answer. Our lives are out of tune with nature. The socialization process, with all its traumas, robbed us of the space to grow up organically. We learned to hurry up. How many times were you told as a child to hurry up? You limited your full inhalation of the breath of life so that you could keep up with the crazy pace of the adults around you.

When you were upset or scared, you held your breath, and you gradually learned that by breathing less deeply you could deaden your feelings. I remember being sad as a child, and lying in bed breathing such small breaths that I imagined I would become invisible and light as a cloud, and I would float away to heaven. It didn't work - I'm still here.

If we had been taught as children to breathe into our feelings instead of holding our breath in times of trouble, our worlds would be different now. Never mind; it is not too late to learn how to breathe.

The majority of us in the western world breathe into our upper chests most of the time. Look around you. Notice your breath and that of the people you spend time with. Notice how people breathe when they are excited, bored, depressed, rushed, overworked, calm, or loving. If you cannot feel your belly moving in and out against your belt as you breathe, then you are breathing into your upper chest.

Only one half cup of your blood circulates through this upper part of your lungs. Your lungs are designed to oxygenate one quart of blood, so you are asking your body to do the work of energizing and detoxifying your entire system on less than one cup of fuel instead of four. Try making a cake with one egg instead of four and see how flat and dense it becomes.

By breathing deeply into your belly, you can function better in this hurry-up world. The paradox is that if we would breathe more deeply, we might have the good sense not to be hurried through our lives. We might slow down to smell the roses and enjoy the pleasures of our senses.

There are special breathing exercises available from many disciplines, and I am going to include here only the three that I like the most and use regularly. This is one of the chapters that requires an investment of time, preferably in the early morning.

Another good time is after work, before you begin your evening activities. If you wait to do the exercise in bed before falling asleep, you may feel calmer, but it is also possible you will feel so full of energy that you may have to get up again. Try it out and find the best timing for yourself. To overcome our unproductive breathing habits, it is important to be regular about this practice.

Rocking Clock Breath

Read through the whole sequence first, then have someone read the instructions to you if possible. Or go online and watch the video on this page – http://comehome2yourbody.com/videos

1. Lie on the floor with your knees up and your feet flat. Imagine, as you lie there, that you are a clock on the wall. At your heart is the number twelve and at your knees is the number six. We will be using this analogy again in a later chapter, so take the time to become familiar with it now. If I were floating on the ceiling above you, looking down, I would see you as a clock face. Your tailbone on the floor is the center of the clock.

2. Now direct your pelvis and belly toward your knees at six o'clock. This is a small movement. Your tailbone does not lift off the floor, but your lower back arches away from the floor and your belly rounds outward. Then rock back and direct your pelvis toward twelve o'clock, at your heart. Your lower back will now press into the floor. Rock gently back and forth between twelve o'clock and six o'clock until you are clear about how this movement feels. Do not work too hard. This is a small and gentle rocking movement. You may know it as the pelvic tilt. You are not pushing with your feet. Your upper back, neck, shoulders, and jaw are fully relaxed.

3. As your belly rounds out toward your knees at six o'clock, inhale a breath deep into your belly. When you are ready to exhale, rock back to twelve o'clock and exhale fully You are breathing at your own rhythm in an easy, unforced way, and the movement of your pelvis is reminding you of where to breathe in and where to breathe out.

   Once that is clear, we will work on the exhalation a little more, since it is the exhalation that is the most important part of this breath. The in-breath will always happen automatically if we wait long enough. The out-breath requires work on the part of the diaphragm, the muscular sheet that separates the lungs from the digestive system.

4. Start to exhale through your mouth as if you were blowing out a candle. (The inhalation is still through the nose.) Exhale completely by pulling your diaphragm up under your ribs. See how much more breath you can exhale when your diaphragm is doing its job. Keep your shoulders

relaxed and don't tighten your buttocks. Notice all the extra muscles you are tensing because you are learning something new. Let them all go.

5. Each time you are completely empty of air, wait until the in-breath comes by itself, deep into your belly. Decrease the effort and blowing of the out-breath until it is soft and gentle and takes twice as long as the in-breath. You are still rocking to remind you where the breath goes. If you try to breathe in when your back is flat against the floor, you will not be able to breath deeply. Let your belly expand and contract. This movement is good for your stomach muscles.

This exercise may sound complicated, but it really isn't. Once you have learned it, practice for five minutes every day to start your day with a sense of balance and personal power. I also recite a mantra in my head on every exhalation. "There is always enough time" is one of my favorites. You can do this breath in bed before you get up, but in the beginning, the hard floor against your backbone makes it easier to learn.

Here is a reminder list:

- Keep your knees up.

- Tilt your pelvis toward six o'clock.

- Arch your back as you breathe into your belly.

- Tilt your pelvis toward twelve o'clock.

40

- Press your back into the floor as you breathe out slowly and fully through rounded lips, pulling your diaphragm up under your ribs.

- Wait for new in-breath to come naturally.

Some Buddhists believe that the space between the breaths is where enlightenment can occur. That space gets longer with this practice, but it has nothing to do with holding your breath. It is a clear moment of no time when you can feel your heartbeat moving through you.

You may have discovered while practicing this exercise that your diaphragm was completely unknown to you. Many of us have allowed our diaphragm to lie around for years on permanent vacation status. By relearning to involve it in our breathing process, we are also helping our digestion. Every internal event in our body happens to its own rhythm, and by allowing your diaphragm to sit out the dance for so long, other parts of you may have become sluggish also. (This may be part of the reason why you pee when you sneeze.)

Through movement of any kind, we encourage all of our autonomic systems—immune, digestive, lymph, endocrine, etc.—to dance to their own rhythms with more energy and aliveness. Can't you just imagine all of these movements inside us, like in a huge dance space where everyone hears their own music and dances to their own tune.

As you continue to practice this exercise for five minutes a day, you may become more aware of your breathing throughout your day. Whenever you do become

41

aware of your breath, take a few deep belly breaths and exhale fully. Very soon, upper chest breathing will feel restrictive to you and will be a sign of tension that will wake you up to your bodily discomfort.

I want to say something about bellies here. Belly breathing may have been deliberately unlearned by us as young women as soon as we became vain. I cannot deny that breathing into your belly will make your belly move in and out. If it doesn't, you aren't doing it correctly. Look at some old pictures of movie stars from the fifties. They all have nice round bellies—Marilyn Monroe, for example. This is normal and healthy.

During my training, there was a lot of joking about a Feldenkrais belly—a belly that moves with the breath, that can give space for digestion, that is strong enough to help support our spine, but never rigid.

Humming Breath

This second breath can be practiced anytime, anywhere. First try to hum on a shallow chest breath. Then hum a tune without thinking about breathing. You will notice that you naturally take a quick belly breath in order to have enough air to hum properly. During the day, whenever you remember, hum a tune you like. This works especially well when you feel yourself tensing up or reacting to your life in a negative way.

Don't let yourself think of reasons why you can't hum. You aren't trying out for the opera. Anyone can hum. It is great for your vocal chords. Allow the sound to drop down from your head to your belly. Hear the different resonances that come from different places in your body. Move the sound up and down between your head and your belly. Have fun with it. Feel all the bones in your head vibrate with the sound. We all resonate to sound on a very deep level. There is a tone exercise in yoga that involves singing, " ooo, eee, aaah, ii, aay, oww," and the tones tune up your whole system. Any vowel will work. If you are tired, this exercise will increase your energy.

Heaven and Earth Breath

This is my favorite. I use it whenever I am out of balance. Read the instructions completely before you start. (There is a lot to learn in this chapter, so take longer than one week if you need to. Practice each breathing exercise and integrate it into your life before you start the next one.)

This is on the same video page here –
http://comehome2yourbody.com/videos

For this exercise, it is best, especially in the beginning, to stand with your feet firmly planted on the earth. That means real dirt if at all possible, not asphalt or concrete. If this is not possible, vividly remember a time when your two feet were planted on the earth. Connecting with the earth seems to be a natural consequence of connecting with our bodies. You may find yourself seeking out nature more often as you become more body-centered.

43

Close your eyes so that you can internalize your attention. If you are nervous about closing your eyes, drop your gaze down to look at your toes. Be comfortable.

Breathe into your belly and imagine that with your in-breath you are pulling energy up from the earth through your feet and up your spine to circle in your heart. Send your out-breath deep into the earth, rooting yourself more firmly in this moment. Imagine what earth energy feels like as it travels through you. It will vary with the seasons and the weather. In the springtime, for me, it is a feeling of new growth, of seeds expanding and pushing up through the darkness, seeking the light. In the summer it feels rich, bursting with abundance. In the autumn there is less pushing upward of this energy; fruits are ready for harvest and the energy is beginning to pull back into the earth. Then in winter, it is a slumbering energy, patiently waiting within the soil for new life.

We are all supported twenty-four hours a day, every second of our life, by the ground beneath our feet, and the force of gravity works to bring us back to the earth in every moment. We can access the living energy and revitalizing power of the earth by breathing in this way. As you breathe this energy up to your heart, imagine a pink light in your heart growing brighter with each breath.

When you have established a deep connection to the earth, let go of your attention to earth energy, knowing it will keep on flowing by itself. Turn your attention now to the sky above your head. With each new breath, bring the energy of Spirit down through the top of your head to your heart. This can be whatever Spirit means to you—heaven, angels, Source, Goddess, God, Infinite Wisdom, the Unknown Mystery—it doesn't care what you call it. This energy is usually lighter, clearer, brighter. I imagine it as an unconditionally loving energy.

As it passes your eyes, affirm that you see clearly with the eyes of love. As it passes your throat, affirm that you speak with loving kindness. As it reaches your heart, let it join the earth energy circulating there, and imagine it making the pink light in your heart even brighter. Your heart may actually *feel* different at this point—bigger, tingling or with a curious ache. Your heart chakra is opening.

Now allow yourself to breathe normally and feel yourself completely balanced, as a channel between Heaven and Earth. You may actually feel a current, like a shimmering pulse, passing up and down your spine as you practice this regularly. With these energies joined inside you, you are limitless. Send the pink light from your heart around your body to any part of you that is blocked or in pain. Imagine it flowing like water. Feel it flow all over your body until your cells dance with aliveness. Then if you choose to, you can send this energy out to anyone in your world who needs it. Imagine it flowing from your heart directly into theirs.

Finally, center back into your own heart and take a moment to appreciate yourself for the wonder that you are. Appreciate yourself for the good that you bring into other's lives. Savor and enjoy this step. Don't rush it.

When you are ready, open your eyes.

After you get used to the Heaven and Earth Breath, complete the whole process in ten breaths—four from earth, four from heaven, and two for healing. The exercise is like making a friend. It takes more time in the beginning, but after a while, just checking in is enough. For me, the Heaven and Earth Breath is a reality check. When I think the world is not giving me what I want, I check in and get back into balance. You may not remember to do it when you need it most at first, but if you practice it regularly, it will become a wonderful tool for balancing and centering.

If you were uncomfortable with this whole process, just skip it. Some people love it and some don't. Many of my clients were embarrassed at first to do anything that invoked Spirit, but I discovered early in my work that without integrating the force of Spirit with body/mind work, deep change was more difficult. There are so many levels to our awareness, and this breath connects us, in a simple way, to some of the deeper levels operating within our psyche.

With any of the inner work or imagination work in this book, the rule is to *fake it 'til you make it.* If you can't possibly imagine earth energy coming up your spine, then just act as if you can. We are all like very exclusive radio receivers. There is an enormous amount of stimuli coming at us at all times and we accept a very narrow range according to our beliefs. We screen out most of it as if it doesn't exist. So allow yourself the freedom to believe that feeling earth energy is possible and you will tune yourself in to the station on which it is playing. We will deal more fully with beliefs and energy in later chapters.

Learn and practice the three breathing exercises and gradually include them in your repertoire, your toolbox of life. This work on your breath is fundamental to a full and happy life. Love yourself enough to practice until breathing correctly becomes a habit.

Moving into this chapter:

Keep writing in your notebook and keep noticing. The chapters are cumulative. Keep noticing from now on.

Practice each of the breaths until they become natural to you.

The Heaven and Earth Breath, especially, will prepare you for the chapter on energy work.

Notice if you get stressed and forget the breathing and if the stress just sticks around or gets worse.

COME HOME TO YOUR BODY

4

FINDING COMFORT

IN SEEKING TRUE COMFORT I FIND PEACE AND JOY

What image does the word comfort bring to your mind? Lounging in a deep armchair in front of a fire, lying on the beach in the sun, hanging out in your robe and slippers, or maybe being held close in loving arms. We all have different images, but for most of us, there will be some slowing down from our normal pace and, probably, some warmth in our picture.

This chapter will allow you to expand your collection of comfort images. I hope to make the definition of that feeling larger in your experience so that you can feel comfort in your body more often and for longer periods of

49

time. When comfort is clear, a feeling of discomfort, instead of pain, can serve as your body's alarm system.

Don't confuse this feeling of comfort with the things we reach for addictively when we are upset, called comfort foods. These are used to numb us to our inner pain and they are just a temporary fix that often has negative long-term consequences.

Can you remember a time when you felt a sense of comfort in doing something you enjoy and do well, without any extra pressure? Pressure of any kind, performance anxiety, drives out comfort and raises our level of stress. Pressure can be external; like time or certain standards that have to be met, or it can be internal; from the high expectations of our inner critic. Wherever the pressure comes from, it erases comfort and pleasure in the task, raises our pulse and our breathing rate, and sets us on edge.

The ideal would be for us to notice those signs of pressure immediately when they first occur in our body and develop a response that allows us to adjust back into comfort. It is by this internal monitoring of our comfort level that we can make adjustments in our lives that lead to increased health and well-being. There is an opinion now amongst researchers that a certain level of stress is good for us. I look at it differently. I would say that we all need challenge; the excitement of new achievement, and the possibility of success, but we don't benefit from discomfort or stress without that challenge.

The first task is to notice what comfort means to you right now. Throughout the day, make a mental note of when you feel content and totally at ease. Comfort can range from a lack of discomfort to undiluted bliss. Notice that.

What about happiness, the goal we are always pursuing? Is happiness the same as comfort for you? What is different about it?

Notice the times when your mouth wants to turn up into a smile for no particular reason. Sometimes when I'm moving along my familiar paths I find myself smiling, and a feeling of joy comes over me just because I am alive on this beautiful earth.

Now start to listen for your specific, internal cues for lack of comfort—your breath, your pulse rate, a feeling of edginess in your jaw, tightness in your stomach or shoulders, a heaviness in your heart, or a urgent need to move away from a situation.

Check your eyes for relaxation, and your hands and feet.

Check the muscles in your neck, shoulders, and belly.

Which cues are the clearest for you?

Anxiety is an extreme on the comfort spectrum.

What do you do when you are anxious?

Do you grind your teeth while you are sleeping?

Do you tap your fingers or feet or bite your nails?

Do you twist your rings or play with your hair or jewelry?

Just notice at this point without trying to change anything.

You are probably very aware, whether you could verbalize it or not, what the body cues are for comfort and discomfort in someone close to you. With one quick glance you can assess the state of mind of your mate, your boss, or your children. Their facial expressions alone probably speak volumes to you. This is a useful skill that women learn through socialization at an early age. I remember, as a child, being fascinated with the changes on the faces of people around me. I could tell exactly how they felt about the people they were with by their minute changes of expression.

Redirect this skill toward yourself. Sneak a look at your own face once in a while, from the inside, without a mirror. You may be surprised at your habitual expression when there is no one else around. Write in your journal a one-word description of what your face conveys. Do you look calm, serene, and happy, or busy, harassed, and troubled? When I did this for the first time I realized that I looked serious a lot. I learned this from my mother. She took life very seriously. So I could be feeling really happy on the inside and yet my grand-kids would ask if I was mad. That was useful feedback!

After a while of noticing you may be disturbed to realize how seldom you are truly comfortable and under what a limited range of conditions. Years ago, when someone first pointed out to me that I was actually a nervous wreck passing as a cool superwoman, I was very surprised. It took a few days for me to accept the truth. I was so high-energy all the time and so busy that I really didn't understand what comfort was. I had to stop my normal behavior of tuning out my body reactions to look for it. My attention had been directed completely toward achievement. I was very results-oriented. I could have said immediately what level of well-being my husband or son were experiencing, because their happiness was on my achievement list, but my own was not. I was surprised to find out that I was living on adrenal energy.

I had an aunt in England who lived on tea and English biscuits—caffeine, gluten and sugar—and I suddenly saw our resemblances. In the same way, a New Yorker friend of mine who visits California, always says after a few days, "Oh no! I'm getting mellow I'd better get back to New York before it's too late." It takes her days to transition into the California lifestyle, but only hours to get sucked back into the energy maelstrom of New York.

It is easier for most people to get hyped up, caught up in stressful circumstances, than it is to unwind. There is a charge of passion and aliveness from dramatic life circumstances that can be addictive. We can become addicted to the adrenaline charge of deadlines and juggling demands. I felt very uneasy at first when exploring comfort because I had to recognize my drama for what it was—an ego defense covering up my discomfort with my life's direction. After a time, you will have a choice about which way you want to go in any moment. Some situations in our lives demand intense energy, but most would really benefit from a deep sense of comfort and peace.

If you find that you are in an anxious, fearful, or upset state, there are specific things you can do to lead yourself back to a greater sense of comfort.

1. If you can lie down, do so. If not, sit in a chair with your back well supported and vertical, both feet on the floor, and your hands separated on your thighs. Breathe deeply into your belly. Move your attention slowly through your body, starting with your toes. Squeeze the muscles in each area as tightly as possible, hold them a moment, and then let go.

   Now put your attention on your heart. Breathe in love from the Universe and breathe out your fear. Set the intention clearly in your mind that you are willing to feel peace in a situation that has bothered you. Notice if you feel comfort with that decision. If not, you may have a desire to continue using the stimulus of the upset for reasons of your own; perhaps to change someone else's behavior. We will deal with that more in the chapter on emotions, but for now see if you can relax into comfort yourself and let the rest of the world be the way it is.

2. Another way to settle into comfort is to relax your face. Our faces hold a lot of tension. They are the windows of our emotional life. Close your eyes and allow your jaw to separate a little. Move your lower jaw in small, slow circles in each direction. Put the middle two fingers of each hand on the joints in front of your ears that move your jaw, the temperomandibular joint. Many of us hold chronic tension at this point. You can find it by opening and closing your mouth. Make small gentle circles with your fingers in this location.

   Then, with your index fingers, make small circles at the space between your eyebrows. Gradually move to other places on your forehead until you have gently massaged your entire forehead. In the same slow, gentle way, with small circles, massage all around your mouth. Now, with all your fingers at once, tap very softly all over your face and neck, making the skin glow.

Lastly, allow your head very gently and slowly to rock back and forth on your neck, looking up to the ceiling and down to your chest. This entire massage process can be done in five minutes and it feels so good.

3. This exercise is for your eyes only. In this culture, we are predominately visual learners. So much of our information comes in through our eyes. I often wonder what cell phones and small electronics are doing to children's eyes. Push your eyes outward as far as they will go, as if your life depended on seeing something written on the wall in very small letters. This is the popeye stare. Notice that your eyes do not work independently. Your jaw, your chin, your neck, and your entire back all tighten up as well.

Now allow your eyes to sink back into your head until your head feels soft and loose on your neck. This is the soft gaze. Look around you with the soft gaze and notice that you can see just as clearly, but it seems as if the world outside is coming to you you are not reaching out to get it.

Go back and forth between the popeye stare and the soft gaze and really become aware of all the differences in the muscles. How far can you trace the tension pattern through your body? When you fully appreciate how tight you feel all over as you reach out with your eyes, you will be able to use your eyes as an indicator for your level of comfort.

We already use this indicator for assessing other people without knowing it. Notice how alarming and upsetting it is to be looked at with the popeye stare and how comforting to be looked at with the soft gaze. As a test, put on your fiercest popeye stare when someone you don't want to talk to approaches you. Use the soft gaze when you want to invite someone's presence. You are a different person when your eyes and face are relaxed.

Releasing Worry

Sometimes I find that my lack of comfort in the moment has nothing to do with what is happening in my life right now. I am busy in my head, either running videos of past pain or worrying about my future. As I move through my day, it can be sunny and peaceful and productive, and yet my past and future voices rob me of my sense of comfort. When I wake up to this, I can center myself back into the moment by breathing into my belly, looking about me with a soft gaze, and appreciating the real, live, concrete goodness in my life right now.

It's amazing how much good we can overlook in the present while we preoccupy ourselves with things that may never happen. If the worry thoughts keep returning, I move my body in ways that bring pleasure—dancing, twirling, or just skipping around the room. Try skipping some time when there is no one around. It never fails to make me feel exhilarated, and I laugh like a child.

For one of my clients who was chronically anxious and depressed, the realization that she had some control over her level of comfort was a point of change. She used to say in the jargon that I call therapese, "I don't feel comfortable with that." What she meant was that she didn't like it or she wouldn't accept it. She finally saw and felt that her life had been a refusal to be comfortable unless she won the changes she wanted from others.

It wasn't working for her. When she made the decision to be comfortable, as a gift to herself, her health improved and her resistance to her world melted away That didn't mean she always liked everything other people chose to do, but she could make her own choices about how to respond without causing herself bodyily discomfort.

In my work there was always a dynamic balance going on between supporting a client and challenging her. Support has a great deal to do with comfort. I made sure she was comfortable because no one learns well in discomfort; but to learn anything new is a challenge. Feldenkrais work is about learning new options, so I constantly seesawed between accepting a client as she was in the moment, and gently leading her to new choices. In my own life it is the same pattern.

You may remember a time in your life when you felt comfortable and supported by your environment and everything was rolling along smoothly. I call these times of grace the plateaus of life. They are resting places of comfort and support for us to prepare for the challenge ahead. Life doesn't seem to allow us to rest on our plateaus for long.

57

Life happens and, ready or not, we are thrust into the next challenge of our growth.

In small ways that you can observe for yourself, there are opportunities to shift from comfort to challenge. Sitting in front of our electronics all evening may seem comfortable in one sense, but it saps our vital life energy. Our bodies get cranky and sluggish when we sit around for too long. For a deeper, truer sense of body comfort, we have to keep moving.

A client, Sandra, came to me about pains in her legs, hips, and lower back. She had a boring job she hated, sitting at a desk all day. She was short, vertically challenged, and her feet didn't touch the floor when she sat in her office chair. That is a strange feeling. I tried it on a high stool and I could immediately feel for myself where her pain was coming from. In the evenings, she would lounge on the couch watching television. She felt as if life were passing her by; as if the stream of her life had slowed and she had washed up in an eddy somewhere covered with green algae.

After we had worked together for a while on her pains and she had adjusted her sitting so that she was supported by her feet, she started to feel more powerful. Within a few months, she had moved within her company to a counter job, dealing with people all day, and she was so much happier she could hardly believe it. Without the pains, she was able to walk on the beach for exercise and she took some classes and met new people instead of watching television. Her body had been trying to tell her something about her life and she finally heard it.

Notice how the people around you react to your level of comfort with yourself. The real you, the person behind the roles you play, is more accessible when you are comfortable. Most people would rather interact with a person than with a role-player. Relationships warm up, there are fewer misunderstandings and trampled feelings, more smiles, and more sincerity.

Notice also how your level of comfort is regularly affected by the people around you. How many people do you know who convey a sense of personal comfort most of the time? Are these people valuable to you? Are they people you feel safe with? Try to spend more time with people who can model this desirable trait for you.

I have a friend who is always a total joy to be around. I have always wished I were more like Lilli. She is upbeat and energetic and lives much of the time in the now moment. People feel better when she is present. My grandmother was the same way. You can probably remember someone in your childhood who made you feel safe and warm.

Imagine what you would do with your body if you wanted a child to feel safe and comfortable with you. What are the small shifts you would make to appear trustworthy to a child. Among other things, you would probably lower your voice, smile, and become totally present. These are sure clues to a feeling of comfort.

In a situation where there are people around you who are anxious or fearful, breathe slowly and deeply into your belly, relax your face, let your eyes rest back into your head, loosen your jaw, and allow a sense of comfort to spread through your muscles. Without saying a word, you are affecting the worried or anxious person for the better. Instead of joining her in her nervous state, you are modeling a more resourceful state. See if you can observe her shift in mood. Having the resource of comfort within is contagious.

Moving into this chapter:

Notice when you are comfortable.

Observe your bodily cues for discomfort.

Observe your habitual expression.

Notice anxiety or distress and do the exercises to relieve it.

Release worry.

Move into a new challenge that excites you.

5

BECOMING A MOVER

I MOVE JOYFULLY TO EXPRESS MY ALIVENESS

C an you remember watching a healthy toddler or small child? They are never still. They run and fuss and wriggle and squirm every second they are awake. Now see if you can remember your first day of school? The school that had desks or tables where you were supposed to sit still for ages and speak only when you were told you could.

How was that for you? Have you buried that memory?

It was in school that we were most firmly socialized into non-movement. Sit still, sit up straight, pay attention, concentrate, no slumping, stop wriggling, no talking, no giggling, take things seriously, do it right. The only person all that control was healthy for was the teacher.

It is way better now than in our childhoods. But, even so, our present educational system is simply *not* a positive environment for learning. It is no wonder that so many of us have trouble with authority figures or with learning new skills. I think it is a tribute to our in-born curiosity and desire to learn and grow that we managed to accomplish as much as we did. Imagine if we had been taught to anchor our mental activity in our bodies. Maybe we would be using a little more of our brains than the five percent we now use.

Dyslexic children have had a lot of success in learning to read by looking at letters repetitively as they bounce on a mini-trampoline. Movement can make us all learn and work better. Prove it for yourself. The next time you have to learn something new, move around a little in a way that is pleasing to you while you are learning. See if you feel more present with the learning experience. You could also try learning two verses of a poem—one while being still and the other while swinging your foot or tapping your fingers. A couple of days later, see what you retain. If you get stuck, repeat the motion you were doing while you were learning.

I have gone to workshops and lectures with people of my own age group, and they sit on hard chairs for hours and barely move a muscle. I can't do it. I have to sit in the back or in the aisle so I can wriggle.

Whenever you have to stand for any length of time, waiting around or waiting in line, get used to moving your body in small ways, almost micro-movements. Travel your awareness through your body from your feet up to your head and see how many muscles you can contract and relax in such small increments that no one notices.

Try it now with your face alone. Our faces are incredibly mobile. Just one small movement can change our expression completely. First see if you can move your facial muscles so slightly that no one can tell. Now try moving as few muscles in your face as possible to change your expression. Try curious, delighted, annoyed, impatient, quizzical, amused, loving, disbelieving, disapproving, satisfied, or any one of your common expressions. I know of a man who spent two years in front of a mirror learning to isolate the movements of his facial muscles. He is a mime and he is incredible to watch.

Now try moving your fingers and toes in the same small way. When you set the intention to move, your muscles respond in microscopic ways. They actually get ready to move before any visible movement is made. First feel the readiness to move, and then move the particular muscle and joint you are using in very small increments in every direction it can go. I have spent more than an hour moving every joint in one hand in every possible way. It's an incredibly relaxing and centering thing to do.

Once you have learned to move in micro-movements, gradually get larger. Wriggle your toes. Shift your weight from one foot to the other. Make circles with one heel at a time. Make circles with one knee at a time. Make some pelvic circles. Tighten one buttock and then the other. Tilt your pelvis by moving your belly forward and back. Then move your ribs in a circle. Shrug your shoulders up toward

63

your ears and let them go. Move your shoulders in circles. Move your wrists and elbows in circles. Move your neck and head in slow, gentle circles. Look down at the floor and up at the ceiling. Look behind you to the right and the left, first with your neck, then with your upper body, and then turning your whole body from your feet.

What you are doing is relearning how to wriggle. When we were impatient children, our wriggling was a sign of repressing larger movements that we were not allowed to make. This time it is our *intention* to make small movements only. Intend the movements to pull your attention back from wherever in the past or future it is wandering, to your body, right now in this moment. This will remind you that you have a body at times when you previously forgot. During your normal working day, when you are caught up in your mind, it is good to check in now and then with your body.

When I was first learning the computer in order to write the first edition of this book, I was very tense and stiff. It was a big change in my life to sit on a chair in one place for any length of time. I was also computer-phobic, which added to my tension. After a couple of days of aches and pains, I came back to my body and realized I needed to wriggle and stretch and let go of mental work at least every half hour. Try it. It will enhance both your productivity and aliveness. If you feel a need to have a full stretch when you become present in your body, then do so. Stretch to the ceiling and then bend down to your toes. Turn sideways from your waist and then stretch out to the side. Make big hula circles with your hips.

Try stretching while waiting in line at the grocery store. Whenever I stretch anywhere, people look at me with approval or envy. Often they will comment and sometimes they will even join in. There is something so luxurious about a full stretch. I think that is why people don't do it very often. It feels too good to do in public. If you are at a board meeting, stick with the micro-movements. No one will notice and it will relieve the tension and the tedium.

Sitting on chairs is cruel and unusual punishment for your body. Also, sitting for long periods in a chair is the worst thing you can do to your back. There is more pressure on your vertebrae while sitting than while doing hard physical labor. In native cultures, most people squat, kneel, or sit cross-legged on the floor, and back problems are rare. Just getting up and down from the floor keeps them healthy.

Right now, see if you can squat easily with your feet fully on the floor. Feldenkrais used to say that this was a sign of good muscular condition and flexibility. When I started my classes, I was surprised by how many people could not squat and could not get up and down from a lying position on the floor. It certainly is true about muscular strength and flexibility that if you don't use it, you lose it. We are restricting our ability to deal with crisis in our lives when our movement is limited in such a way. Ideally, we should be able to move quickly in any direction—up, down, forward, back, and sideways.

If this is difficult for you because of pain you have to be aware that the cycle of pain and stiffness is a very vicious circle. If you have pain, you stiffen up; if you stiffen up, you have more pain. The longer my mother spent sitting during the day instead of moving about, cooking, shopping, and gardening, the stiffer she got. The increasing amount of time spent sitting nowadays in this culture adds enormously to the epidemic of back problems.

Another problem caused primarily by too much sitting is the loss of bladder control. If our chairs are usually supporting all of the organs of our lower body, the muscles of the perineum give up their work of holding them all in place. If you have a problem with bladder control when you sneeze, cough, or laugh, take heed of the warning signals.

The most helpful thing I have found is to get a small rebounder. They are mini trampolines, and the gentle bouncing works to strengthen all the muscles in the pelvic floor. I have one beside my desk and I love it. Jumping up and down to one or two favorite songs reawakens my body, shakes the cobwebs out of my brain, and helps all my internal organs function better. It is the best quick exercise break I know. There should be one in every office.

When you start bouncing, you may find that you have to stop and go to the bathroom at almost every bounce at first. Start out with a very small movement of raising your heels only, so that both feet are always on the mat, and graduate up to jumping and jogging. Within a week, your muscles will have strengthened noticeably.

If you *have* to sit for long periods of time at work, remind yourself to get up and walk around and stretch every half-hour. Even as you are sitting you can get into the habit of bending and arching your spine. Fold your spine by bringing your chin toward your thighs and then look up toward the ceiling, arching your spine as much as is comfortable. Do the same bending and arching movement some more, but orient your body to the right a few times, and then to the left. Can you feel each vertebra along your spine joining in one at a time, or are you moving in three chunks? The more often you do this the more articulated your spine will feel. Finish up with some pelvic circles while sitting in your chair.

Stretch your spine when you get up in the morning by sitting on the edge of the bed and making all of these movements.

The pelvic circles, especially, will free up your spine for the day ahead. If you wake up stiff, make very small and slow circles at first.

Instead of sitting on chairs and couches at home, try sitting on the floor for a week. You could also try squatting to watch television and see how long you can be comfortable in this position. I often sit on the floor because I am freer to move from there. You can roll around and bend and stretch in all kinds of ways that are impossible in a chair. You may be stiff the first day, but by the end of the week you will almost certainly feel looser and more flexible.

It would be hard to do most of our jobs while squatting, unfortunately, so the best way to sit at your desk is with both feet planted firmly on the floor. In that position, your spine can be erect with its natural curves and there are four points of support—your two feet and your two sitz bones. If you sit far back in your chair and lean on the backrest, you are giving up the task of supporting your body with your spine. The chair takes over the job. When you are relaxing completely that is fine, but when you are working it is not a good idea.

When you lean on the back of your chair and extend your arms to work—writing, typing, etc.—you develop shoulder stiffness and tension. We are designed to move from the strong muscles of the pelvis and feet, and to use the articulation of all of the vertebrae. By constraining this area in the chair, we cause our neck and shoulders to do more work than they were designed to do.

There is no perfect ergonomic chair on the market that will negate the necessity to move and to wriggle. Actually, it is better to change chairs often, just as it is better for your feet to change shoes during the day. There is no one perfect position we can settle into and be safe. From the perspective of design, we were not well-designed for a sedentary lifestyle at all. We were designed to move and then to rest completely between movements – like a cat.

I built a standing desk for my computer work when I began getting pains in my neck and shoulders from leaning forward while typing and reading. I love it and I custom designed it for my height and the length of my arms. Now I can type for hours and never have shoulder pain. I also cut down my browsing time because it's less comfortable to stand and browse for hours.

Many of the movements we learned in physical education class are very straight-line in design—jumping jacks, for example. When we use circular motions, with our spine as the axis, our movements are more natural and easier on the body. Imagine a dancer in your mind and see all the circular movements common to most dance forms. When you are moving through your daily tasks alone, pretend you are a dancer. Make your movements bigger, rounder, more graceful. Reach with your whole body from your toes instead of from your overworked shoulders. Bend all the way down, making sure not to lock the knees, whenever you need to bend.

Imagine a flow of movement instead of jerky, short, sudden moves. Put on some music and see how flowing you can be. Notice if you have a tendency to use your neck alone whenever you need to look at something to the side or behind you. Turn your whole body instead. We get so accustomed to overworking our arms, legs, and neck, and leaving our trunk rigid. Our spines are articulated like a bicycle chain; they turn, they bend, they stretch.

While you are walking around the house, think tall and light, and incorporate a few leaps and jumps and runs into your day. It is always good to have those skills available. My sister, Diane, was visiting me from England some years ago and we were crossing a street with cars waiting when the "Don't walk" sign came on. Naturally I started to run, but when I called out to her to do the same, she walked at her normal pace. She said, "I don't run for anything" in a disapproving tone as if she were way too old for that kind of silly behavior. She was totally rigid and not yet fifty.

It was frightening to me how easily she could make a virtue out of being stiff and tight. I made up my mind right then that I would run and jump and skip and climb trees

69

until I died. Not all the time, of course, but often enough so I wouldn't forget how. We have to be willing to be childlike on occasion to remember the pure joy of just being in our body, playing at life. We get too serious about being grownups. It's just a role we play. We don't have to lose ourselves in it. So put away all your chairs, roll around on the floor, and wriggle a lot. Your spine, neck, shoulders and, in fact, your whole body will be grateful.

Moving into this chapter:

Try all the movements described in the chapter until you start to become involved in the exploration with a sense of curiosity. Then make up a million more.

Stop sitting whenever possible.

Move vigorously every hour at least.

Wherever you are, WRIGGLE!

6

HABITUAL PATTERNS

I HAVE CHOICE IN EACH MOMENT

Habitual patterns are those things we do without thought, except to wonder at times why everybody else doesn't do the same thing. These patterns usually have both a physical and a psychological or emotional component. There are habitual patterns that are cultural, such as being friendly toward strangers; there are habitual patterns that are gender differentiated, such as women being ready to give comfort when someone looks upset; and there are idiosyncratic patterns you have that you think are the norm; such as finishing other people's sentences, but that drive your friends wild.

71

This week, we are going on the hunt for these habitual patterns in ourselves and others. Once again, the object of the game is to have choice. If our habits are running us without our awareness, we don't have choice.

One of the major premises in this book is that the more we learn about ourselves and the more options that are available to us, the richer our lives will be. If we see the brain as an incredibly complex network of connections, anything new we learn creates a new neural pathway. Instead of traveling on the old, rutted paths of our habitual patterns, we will be striking out and making new tracks within our brain, which will be available to us forever.

Usually, we notice patterns in our daily lives only when someone remarks on them. Otherwise, we go merrily on our way thinking we are the same as everyone else. When a person comments on our habitual optimism, or our way of interrupting all the time, or our habit of looking for the best in people, we become aware that we are different. We look at the world in our own special way.

An easy way to discover some of your habitual patterns for yourself is to notice whenever you say, "I always" or "I never." Both of these statements are limitations, and that is what most habits are. It saves us time to have habits. If we had to be fresh and new in every moment, we would never get anything done; but habit also limits our experience.

Being territorial is a very common human pattern. We stake out our claim to a certain chair or spot and get upset when others don't realize it is ours. That reminds me of the women in Las Vegas who play the slot machines. They lay claim to a whole row of slots and you could suffer grievous bodily harm if you put a quarter in one of *their* machines by mistake.

Another way to bring your own patterns to awareness is to notice when you are surprised or shocked by someone else's behavior. Obviously, their pattern is different than yours, and your own is so familiar to you that you think it is universal. You also probably think it is *right!*

In England, when I grew up, there was consensus about many of our daily behaviors. We all learned early the *proper* way to do everything and the social perils of deviation. In the wonderful melting pot of ethnic groups here in the United States, there is less conformity to tradition and more freedom to discover new patterns for ourselves. Trying something new could even be said to be an honored American pattern.

We have many purely physical habits that are so ingrained we are unaware of them: the way we walk and talk and laugh, for example. Usually, any member of a family can tell which other family member is approaching from the sound of their footsteps alone. Science has discovered that it is not only our fingerprint that can identify us beyond doubt, our voiceprint is also unique. Even within a family, our voices are all usually very dissimilar. The way we hold our jaw to speak is the result of our own particular view of the world. Some habits can be changed as soon as they are brought into awareness and others cannot. We can change our accent with a little work, but our unique voice-print will still give us away.

73

One physical pattern I changed recently was squinting in the sun. I was getting a crease, like a frown, between my eyebrows and starting to look like a grouch, so I quickly learned not to squint. As we get older, the lines on our faces tell a story about our lives, through our habitual patterns of expression.

Gravity is a mixed blessing as we age. As our mouths start to droop toward our feet, it takes a very optimistic outlook on life to look habitually cheerful. If, indeed, we would even want to.

What does your habitual expression say about you?

One of the most prominent physical habit patterns is our choice of right or left hand dominance. Feldenkrais thought that if we would become ambidextrous, we would be adding an enormous new capacity to the brain.

Try doing some less important tasks with your non-habitual hand this week, maybe brushing your hair or teeth. It may feel awkward at first, but it could help to equalize the wear on your wrist and shoulder joints as well as create new pathways in your brain.

Have you noticed that most people hold one shoulder higher than the other? Figure out for yourself which shoulder is higher on most people, the shoulder of their dominant hand or the other one.

We also have a dominant standing leg. We stand with most of our weight on one leg most of the time, and we usually move out first with the other leg. We choose to jump or climb steps with the moving leg first. See if you can alternate legs and stand with your weight on your

74

moving leg more. You will gradually come to feel more balanced.

As people become upset or anxious, the first physical habitual pattern to kick in will be breathing into their upper chest. If the anxiety continues, you will notice all kinds of unconscious worry movements—biting their nails, compulsive eating, scratching, shaking, twitching, tapping hands or feet, etc. When people are happy and content, these behaviors are absent.

Are you habitually late or early for every appointment? Do you often go out with someone who is the opposite? This is a surprisingly frequent cause of disagreements.

Notice which is your habitual preference without making it good or bad. Experiment with changing. If you are always early, pick an occasion when you won't drastically affect anyone else, and try to arrive late. You may find this very difficult at first. Persist until you manage it, even if you experience some anxiety.

This is an old childhood pattern, and the reason for the anxiety usually has little to do with the present. The young age at which this pattern was learned is the reason it polarizes people so much. Our parents and teachers always wanted us to be on time and we were punished in various ways for being late. Some of us are complying tenaciously and some of us are still rebelling thirty years later.

If you are a habitual late-comer, give yourself permission to stop the rebellion and try being early. Once again, you may find it astonishingly difficult. People I know trick themselves with fast clocks or leave with time to burn,

75

and still somehow manage to arrive late. Notice your feelings about it. Are you irritated that people get so hung up about time? Is it depressing to always be upsetting people with your lateness? Go back and forth between being early and late and see what feels comfortable for you. Bring the whole pattern into conscious awareness.

I am an early bird partly because I am usually eager to get on with life. If its good, let me at it. If its bad, let's get it over with. After experimenting for a while, I felt that I had a choice. When I am late now I don't get anxious about it. I sometimes even choose to be late for certain events, especially in California. When I arrived on time, I often found my hostess in the shower or I was enlisted to help cook dinner.

Another side benefit of this experiment is that I no longer get angry when other people are late. I used to think they were inconsiderate and rude, and I took it very personally when they were late. Now I just do what I need to do—leave without them or wait without rancor.

There are many gender-specific patterns that have a psychological component as well as a physical one. A very common pattern with women concerns helping. *We are just such helpful people!* When I had a male client for Feldenkrais work or massage and I picked up an arm or a leg, they generally lay there like the dead and let me get on with it. Not so with women. As soon as I reach out to pick up their arm, there it is in my hand. As soon as they think they know where I am going to go with it, there it is.

In Feldenkrais, it is important to not help, to be a passive learner, but it is no use saying that at first. Women have a hard time *not* helping. Its a new skill and they have to learn it. This deeply ingrained pattern is important to examine because some of us get so little true rest. Even if no one needs anything at the moment, we are on the alert on a subconscious level for when they do.

It was very common among English women when I grew up, that as soon as a desire escapes the lips of her husband or children, she is on her way to gratifying it. If their loved ones don't speak up, they will constantly ask, "Does anyone want a cup of tea? Is anyone hungry? Don't you need a sweater?" Maybe it is more common in England, but I have seen it often enough here in the United States also.

A good time to notice this pattern is at mealtimes. If you are sitting at the table and a member of your family wants something, do you jump up and get it? Are you always asking your family if there is anything they want or need? Are you genuinely happy to be of service in these small ways, or are you often resentful?

It is often not a positive thing to do tasks for others that they could do for themselves. The help comes from a loving heart, but it does not encourage self-reliance. A friend of mine never taught her children to take a share in the household chores when they were small. Now they are teenagers and she can't wait for them to grow up and leave. They take her work of making their home comfortable completely for granted.

The point is that your body will wear out sooner if you are constantly ready to act on others whims; In answering our own desires, our bodies can fully relax between the movements we make to satisfy these desires. That is the way our bodies were designed, to move and to rest fully between movements. When we are at the beck and call of others, this complete relaxation no longer occurs.

When I asked one client, who was very stiff, to watch for the helping habit in her life, she replied that she had no children and a loving husband, and she did not have that pattern. During the next week, she was surprised to discover that she certainly did. It would be unusual for a woman not to have it after the socialization of so many centuries. Look for this pattern in your own life this week.

In addition to the helping pattern, we have many other habitual patterns that are gender differentiated. Of course, we are all a blend of feminine and masculine energies, and many women have a lot of male patterns in their repertoire. In fact, we have been encouraged since the women's liberation movement to acquire common male patterns in order to make it in the business world. Being competitive, being linear, and following rules are patterns common to men that women have had to learn.

When men and women are complaining about each other, we can notice some opposite patterns. Women will say men are inflexible, while men will say women are too changeable. Women say men are non-verbal, while men say women talk too much. Once again, the peaceful solution is to recognize and celebrate our differences. Who would want to live in a world full of clones?

Think of a feminine pattern you have, and try not to get caught up in it this week. For example, are you a comforter? Do you need everyone in your world to be happy and content all the time? Do you mediate all the quarrels and comfort the wounded? Are you a woman people can count on to make *their* troubles your own? Do you ignore your own need for comforting?

Try putting yourself first for a week. Allow people their unhappiness. No one can be happy all the time. This is a world of duality. Too much of the same emotion is boring. Accepting someone's negative feelings without trying to help them or change them is a real gift. What you learn about yourself will be interesting.

Nurturing, cleaning, caring, sympathizing, cooking, picking up after, helping, finding, comforting, joining, sharing, being efficient, mediating, remembering, being spontaneous, intuitive, and sensitive are some feminine patterns. Many of them are actually the skills of a homemaker, and a lot of younger women have fewer of these patterns, if any. Probably because they had working mothers.

We all have hundreds of habitual patterns we can pay attention to. It is funny how just recognizing them often makes us feel better. I used to feel very upset when my second husband and I had a silly fight after a period of intense closeness. I finally realized that it was a habitual pattern of his to create distance in that way when we got too close. When we brought it out in the open, we no longer needed to fight. He would just say that his bliss

79

tolerance level had been exceeded and he needed some space.

If a close friend has a pattern you don't have, try it out. Pick a positive pattern at first, something like jumping out of bed wide awake and happy. It's odd how we don't think we have choice about something like that. Then try the opposite, pushing the snooze button ten times, snuggling back under the covers, refusing to think about the day ahead, and finally getting up at the last minute. See which pattern works better for you.

I had a sleep pattern for years that required absolute quiet and darkness before I could sleep. It was a real bother. I didn't realize back then that I could change it. I thought that was just the way I was. Fortunately, I was smart enough to teach my son, Tim, to sleep anytime, anywhere. I finally outgrew my pattern on a year-long trip to South America under somewhat grueling conditions. On that trip, if I hadn't given up the need for quiet and darkness, I would never have had a good night's sleep. By the end of the trip I could sleep on buses, trains, restaurant seats, hard beds, even next door to a riotous celebration.

Now I have the same pattern as Tim; when I am tired, I sleep wherever I am. Life is so much simpler. What we have to remember is that we all have a list of preferences a mile long and we often create habitual patterns around them. Just remember that you created your preferences and your habits, and you can change them if they no longer suit you.

80

Now if you are ready for a challenge, pick a habitual pattern a friend has that has always bothered you. Explore the pattern for yourself. Not with a feeling of vengeance—I'll show her how it feels—but with a desire to learn. The pattern obviously works for her on some level; maybe you can learn from it.

Unreliability has always been one of my biggest aggravations. What I learned from my exploration was the sweet sense of freedom I could feel when I forgot everyone else's plans and needs. It was such a carefree feeling at first. I knew that my friend didn't do it on purpose to irritate me. She is just better at forgetting than I am. I finally came to realize that I had always been painfully super-conscientious. Of course, I always subconsciously expected a payoff for my goodness and got very resentful when no one noticed.

I learned a lot from exploring many facets of unreliability, but after a while, I decided that the pattern didn't feel natural for me. I didn't feel as connected as before. The good part is that I no longer get irritated with my friend for having that pattern. I am now more willing to double check our arrangements with her in case she forgets. Another funny thing is that I seemed to be surrounded by people who were unreliable and forgetful before, and now, if I am, I don't notice it.

You have probably noticed by now that many of our habitual patterns occur in pairs—early bird/late-comer, reliable/ unreliable, etc. In relationships, and within families, it is not coincidental that most conflict occurs around these polarities.

81

It is almost as if we internally decide which roles we will play when we first meet. "Okay, I'll take dependent, but you have to take authoritarian, and you can take moody too. I'll be merrily empty-headed and you can be serious."

Sometimes this division of roles can last a long time, but eventually, one of the partners changes and upsets the balance. Then the unspoken negotiation has to start all over again.

Examine your life with total honesty and see if you can decide which side of some of these polarities you are on:

Giver/receiver
Shy/outgoing
Introvert/extrovert
Meticulous/careless
Obedient/rebellious
Tactful/outspoken
Child/parent
Rational/intuitive
Affectionate/cold
Honest/dishonest
Loose/tight
Optimistic/pessimistic
Winner/loser
Pleaser/rebel
Clever/stupid

With different people in our lives, we often act out different sides of the polarity. We will probably act in a different way around men than among women. If you act like a winner with some people and like a loser with others, ask yourself what it is about the relationship that evokes that behavior from you.

Notice if you have a strong reaction to one of the polarities, dishonesty for example. Most of us would like to think that we are honest women, but I'm certain there is some small corner of your life in which you are less than totally truthful. The value of this experiment is to discover for ourselves that we can be anything we choose, if only for five minutes.

Pick one polarity that you are used to playing and act out its opposite. Other people will have to adjust their behavior and they may resist and try to force you back into the old pattern. To experience the new pattern successfully, you have to feel in your belly how it would feel and then allow your body to act it out. A loser has different body posture than a winner. If you forget how the role feels, go back to your belly and imagine being in the role until it starts to come naturally.

This may not be easy. You may think you can't possibly be gregarious; you are shy and that's all there is to it. Not true. You have been around gregarious people and have seen this trait modeled, so somewhere in your body/mind that pattern is ready to be expressed. Your body/mind knows more than you can possibly imagine. You are truly unlimited in the roles you can play, so go ahead and audition for some new choices. Have fun with this exercise.

Habitual patterns are usually based on beliefs we hold about reality. We aren't always conscious of our beliefs, but

83

they form the underpinnings of our behaviors. Imagine that you are describing yourself to someone. Write a description in your notebook. Start with I am …. For example: I am a quick thinker, a morning person, somewhat reserved, often moody, etc.

Everything you wrote is a belief you hold about yourself. Have you ever had a belief about yourself that changed drastically? I used to say I had no musical aptitude. I wished I did, but I didn't, just like I don't have green eyes. Lately I have been taking a course on speaking and singing and finding out that I can do both. I love it!

Any belief can be changed. We change an enormous number of beliefs about ourselves as we grow up. Think of some beliefs you had about yourself as a teenager that you just grew out of. I believed for years as a pre-teen and young teenager that I would never get a date. Here I am two ex-husbands later.

Most beliefs, like the habitual patterns they create, limit us in some way. I decided long ago to choose some primary beliefs for myself that give me more freedom.

I believe I am limited only by my interests. That means I'll never be like Georgia O'Keefe or Beethoven because I am not willing to put all my time and energy into art or music; but whatever interests me I can learn and do well.

My life is a journey guided by Spirit. The habitual pattern that comes out of this belief would be learning from everything that happens to me whether it feels good or bad at the time.

Think of beliefs, and the habitual patterns that come from them, as the roles you have chosen for yourself, or that maybe your parents chose for you. In the hypothetical example of being somewhat reserved, the habitual pattern of behavior would be to hang back, not join in, not smile much, not be open and forthcoming, not trust people readily, and to be cautious. Do you see how limiting that is? If all our life is but a stage, as Shakespeare said, maybe we would want to play that role for a while to see how it feels, but surely not forever!

Go back to the description you wrote about yourself and look at the roles you are choosing to play. If some of the roles are too limiting for you, pick some new beliefs, try out some different habitual patterns, and write your own script.

This *is your life, you get to choose.*

Moving into this chapter:

Notice when you say, "I always...or I never..."

Try doing some tasks with your non-dominant side.

Stop helping and put yourself first.

Discover your polarities and explore the opposite.

Explore beliefs and change them if they no longer serve you.

COME HOME TO YOUR BODY

7

WALKING IN YOUR WORLD

I WALK FORWARD INTO MY LIFE WITH AN OPEN HEART

To walk with freedom and grace in our world demands both muscular, mechanical skills and a psychological and spiritual connection with that world. We are the first member of the animal kingdom to choose to walk erect. By doing so we expose our soft bellies, genitals, and hearts to the rest of the world and to each other. This is a very vulnerable position. To walk forward confidently, we need to feel safe within our vulnerability.

How many people do you know who have a walk that telegraphs peace and personal power to all who see it? It's rare, isn't it? Usually it comes with the self-acceptance of maturity, if at all. That kind of confidence is also environment-specific for most of us. We will walk more freely in our own home territory than in a strange place. There is, however, a sense of safety and centeredness that we can learn to carry within us.

Einstein said that you could divide people into two groups—those for whom the world is a safe place and those for whom it is not. That personal sense of safety comes from the acknowledgment of our connections, both to the Universe and to each other. If we see most of the people in our world as well-loved sisters, brothers, and friends, we can negotiate for our needs with ease.

It is when we feel we have potential adversaries or enemies in the environment around us that we lack trust and hold our breath and tighten up. We retreat to a small safety zone in our minds somewhere and leave our bodies alone out there in the world to take care of themselves as best they can. This is when we become clumsy and uncoordinated and move like puppets. It is a very clear indication of our mental state when we move in this way. Most accidents happen when we are completely entangled in our mental processes and not in our bodies at all.

Taking all of these factors into account, walking becomes a complex topic. I will divide the movements into segments for you to notice in yourself. I have included certain practical suggestions that can lead to better health and range of motion in your entire body. Underlying all of them are the psychological implications of the movements themselves, and the personal history of your very particular way of walking in your world. It is impossible to separate the two. By walking differently we become different.

Feldenkrais believed that learning to move in a new effortless way would change our lives completely. That was certainly true for me. Here is just one small example. I had a pattern of locking my knees that I was unaware of. I just knew that I couldn't learn to ice skate or ski or do anything that required balance. I felt inadequate because of that. It was a limitation in my self-image. During my Feldenkrais training I had a hands-on session of Functional Integration and my knees became more pliant. It was impossible to explain, but they just didn't need to lock anymore. As I walked in this new way, I recaptured memories of my childhood that had been locked in my cells.

As a toddler, whenever I got to my feet my older sister would push me down. I tried to hold on to the floor by curling my toes under and locking my knees. This was the opposite of useful because locked knees make us more unstable, but what does a baby know about body mechanics? So many of our decisions to be, to move, to act in a certain way, are made before we have any logical thought processes operating. We move toward pleasure and away from pain in the natural way of kittens, and make decisions that often last a lifetime.

When I was able to let go of locking my knees in response to stress, I moved into a bigger version of who I was, I became more fully the person I was born to be. In the process of moving in a new way, you may discover for yourself where your limitations began.

89

Whether you remember the specific details is not important. We have all been guided into a very limited path of expression by our socialization. Most of the time we seem locked into either blind acceptance or resistance to our early role models. For all of us, there are so many paths not taken. By learning to move differently, we discover choices that we never before imagined were available to us.

Let's check your habitual posture or state of alignment. Stand as you would while waiting in line at the store and notice yourself from your toes to your head, as completely as possible.

Now stand with your feet apart, the same width as your hips, so that your feet are directly underneath you. Balance evenly between them with your knees unlocked and your spine straight. Let your arms hang freely at your sides. Your head and eyes face the horizon. Breathe deeply into your belly.

How do you feel? This direct, forward-facing position is very exposed, isn't it? We rarely stand like this. We normally shift our weight or do something with our arms to cover our exposed frontal surfaces.

From this balanced position, gradually round your upper back so your shoulders slump forward. Feel your knees bend a little and your neck compress and let your eyes drop to the floor ahead of you. Your arms will hang in front of your thighs.

How do you feel now?
Are you depressed yet?
Who does this remind you of?

Walk around like this and notice if your arms can swing.

Do you drag your feet?
Do you stare at the floor ahead?

This is the home position of someone who is saying NO to life. It is also a common position of elderly people. This is not a necessary posture of old age. We are choosing how we look at eighty by our movement patterns all our lives and by our daily reactions to life's inevitable sorrows and disappointments.

Come back to the balanced position and breathe deeply. Now put your finger on your breastbone between your breasts and push that part of you forward, up and out. Your back will arch, your knees will start to lock, your buttocks will tighten, your chin will come forward, and your aims will hang behind your thighs. Your hands may tend to clench into fists. Your shoulder blades will come closer to your spine.

How do you feel?
Who does this remind you of?

Stride around like this for a while. Get into it, especially if this body posture is completely foreign to you.

This is the home position of someone with an aggressive approach to life. They are using muscular armor to hide their vulnerability. Their body language says, "Don't mess with me." Underneath that they are usually saying, "I'm scared and confused so I'm trying to look tough."

Come back to your own habitual posture. Where does it fall on this huge range? What are you saying to the world? There are endless variations:

I am friendly or leave me alone.
I am better than you or pity me.

I had a client who stood before me when we met with her hands clasped in front of her, one foot leaning on the other and her head bent down a little so that she was looking up at me with her eyes. She had a neck problem that was persistent and could not be diagnosed. No wonder!

Try that position for yourself. It is the position of a child in a world of unreliable adults. After changing her way of standing, walking, and moving, she started to reclaim her power. She is more assertive now and no longer sees almost everyone in the guise of an authority figure. She was even able to be open and firm with a family member who had previously abused her. We cannot change our past, but with movement we can create choice in our present.

Starting with the Feet

Now we will start back at the bottom, with our feet. Our feet are miraculous. They are designed to move. They have twenty-six bones and thirty-one joints. They are not designed for high-heeled shoes or for the flat, hard surfaces we encounter all day long. In Africa and the Ancient Americas, certain tribes could run all day on rough, uneven terrain without shoes and without tiring. The best thing you can do for your feet is to take off your shoes as often as possible and walk barefoot on uneven surfaces. I grew up in a seaside town with a pebble beach and we locals always laughed watching tourists trying to walk on the pebbles. We could run on them easily, from much practice; maybe that is why my feet are so healthy today. Now I wear minimalist footwear when I have to and have bare feet whenever possible. I *never* wear shoes with any heel at all.

Many of my clients have extremely sensitive feet that act as if they have only two joints. It is hard to persuade these clients to walk barefoot, even on a soft rug; but without full utilization of all the joints of our feet, there is no way for us to move freely.

The second thing you can do to benefit your feet is to move them in every way you can think of, both on and off the ground. Turn, twist, bend, stretch, and rotate. When you are sitting reading or watching television, allow your feet to explore their possibilities.

My son, Tim, had something wrong with his feet as a child and was prescribed plastic supports for his shoes. They didn't improve anything. Then he took up surfing, which is an intricate dance between your feet and the ocean, and his feet never bothered him again.

Walk around for a while without shoes and feel how your feet contact the floor. Walk on the inside of your feet and notice what that does to your knees. Then try walking on the outside edge of your feet. Notice that even a small inward or outward slant to your feet will put your knees and hips out of alignment.

Now stop walking on the floor as if it were just a dead surface and walk as if you were walking on the earth. Feel the energy of the earth rise up to support you. Make walking an interaction between you and the earth, no matter how many layers of concrete there are between you. Have you ever walked on a floating bridge? There is a dynamic interaction between your feet and the water. Imagine that the earth interacts with your feet in the same way, but more subtly.

Walking with connection to the earth gives us power. If you have been doing the Heaven and Earth breath regularly, you will have experienced that by now. If you press into the earth more with the balls of your feet so that your feet bend at each step, you will be able to walk longer with less fatigue. When I walk on the beach with a friend and we are talking, my awareness is focused on my mind and my feet get tired. When I am present in my body and pushing off of the balls of my feet at each step, I can walk for miles.

Our hamstrings are the strong muscles at the back of our legs that are supposed to do most of the work of walking. By the time we are thirty, many of us have learned how to ooze along somehow without activating them. Stand with your feet hip-width apart and push into the ground with the ball of your left foot; your heel will rise slightly Notice the motion traveling up your leg and into your behind. The harder you push, the more of your powerful walking muscles get involved. Now try the right foot.

94

Walk around and allow these muscles—the hamstrings and the gluteal muscles of your buttocks—to spring into action at each step. Tighten them consciously at first. You may look like those men who do walking races. You will either get taller at each step or move forward faster. Practice until you can walk with or without the work of these muscles and know how different it feels. When you have to walk a long way or you are in a hurry, actively involve these muscles. Your bottom will become firmer as a side benefit from walking in this way. Your hips will also rotate more, which will be good for your lower back.

I am not including a section on knees because problems with the knees do not generally originate there, except in the case of accidental injuries. Most knee problems originate in the hips or the feet. For women of my mother's generation, hip and knee replacement surgeries are becoming commonplace, and I have been wondering whether we baby-boomers will be the same. There is a much greater awareness of the value of exercise now, but overall, our lives are more sedentary than ever.

A huge factor in the wear on hip joints that makes a hip replacement necessary is poor body alignment. I am sorry to say that, in general, my age group seems to have even worse alignment than my mother's. The number of children with poor alignment is also increasing enormously as so many kids sit in front of televisions or electronics instead of moving around playing.

Our hips are ball and socket joints. A lot of women move as if they don't know that. They act as if their hip joints are hinge joints like their knees. Stand up and hold onto something lightly for support and put your finger on your hip joint. It is located in the middle of the crease between your crotch and your hip-bone. Now bend your knee like a hinge and then bring your bent knee up toward your chest. That action uses your hip joint like a hinge.

Now take your knee in circles in every direction that is comfortable—side, up, down, back. You can do that only because your hip is a ball and socket joint. It's a miraculous piece of engineering and makes the wonder and beauty of dance possible.

Walk around for a while without allowing your hip joint to rotate. Your whole trunk must face forward and your hip joints will act like your knee joints. This is the walk of the wooden soldier or of a woman who has been raised to keep her bottom still as she walks. I am sure that this restriction in walking has a lot to do with the many hip problems experienced by my mother's generation. In Italy and France, women walk in a sensuous, hip-swinging way and hip replacement surgeries are uncommon.

Now walk letting your bottom move freely. In fact, exaggerate, walk like a movie star. Wiggle that behind. Notice how your hips are rotating beautifully. Notice how freely your upper body moves and your aims swing. This is a walk that involves more of you. It is more healthy in general. Tone down the wiggle until you can still feel the rotation in your hips, but it is discreet enough for your taste. Actually it is a pleasure to see people walk with their hips moving freely, and it doesn't look as provocative as it feels at first.

96

The next time you are hurrying along with your mind going at a faster clip than your feet, notice what part of your body seems to be leading the rest. I used to catch myself leaning far forward like a speedskater and bustling here and there as if my mind were dragging my body along. It isn't efficient! If you are in a hurry, push off with the balls of your feet, activate your most powerful muscles, and stay in your body. You will get where you are going even sooner and more safely.

If you imagine a string tied to your belly button and someone pulling on the string as you walk, you will be leading your movement from a good place of balance. Don't stick your belly out, they aren't pulling the string that hard. Center your attention at that point as you walk and the self-confidence we were talking about at the beginning of the chapter will start to kick in. This is the point of Chi in martial arts, and it is the point around which we can rotate in any direction. It is our physical center. The powerful muscles of the pelvis and lower back are all working in harmony, leaving your upper body free to do other work.

When I see people power walking for exercise, pumping away with their arms and upper body, holding visible tension in their shoulders and neck, leaning forward and gritting their teeth, I want to beg them to stop. Let your feet, legs, and the powerful muscles in your bottom do your walking and let every muscle above them be loose and free and along for the ride. Your arms will swing freely by themselves if your hips are rotating and your lower back is moving. There is no need for tension in your shoulders or neck as you walk. A good test of a healthy walk is the ability to leap into the air freely at any time without any planning or preparation.

Pretty soon you will be walking so freely that you will leap into the air and spin and turn just for the sheer joy of it. Being in a body that can move is a pleasure beyond reckoning. We lose it so gradually, if indeed we ever had it, that we never mourn the loss. Regain that pleasure for yourself right now. You have to walk around anyway, you may as well delight in it.

Moving into this chapter:

Try the YES and NO standing positions and see where you fall on the continuum.

Take your shoes off and wriggle your feet.

Throw your high heels away, they are killing you.

Use your glutes in your bottom when walking.

Allow your hip joints full range of motion.

8

MOVING INTO SELF-LOVE

I LOVE MYSELF AS THE UNIVERSE LOVES ME

Self-love was not a buzzword 16 years ago when I first wrote this book. I didn't give much thought to it then. I probably would have said I loved myself well enough at the time but that would have been far from true. I was still caught up in trying to please others. I had not yet realized that I was an empath; someone who feels the feelings of the people she is around. I think most women have this quality but, for some of us, it is powerful enough to give us a desperate need to keep everyone in our lives happy.

If you can walk into a room and be able to tell immediately who in the room is sad or angry or happy, then you are an empath also. It's a tough card to pull. For most of my life I didn't like to be in large groups or in groups that were drinking or doing drugs, and I thought I was unsociable, a party-pooper. When I got sick I became a virtual hermit until I had worked my way gradually back to health. Even now I prefer my own company more often than not, given the present vibration of lack and fear so prevalent in the world.

Self-love, for me, is being willing to say no to others when I need to. To be able to withstand the emotions I feel from them about not getting their way, and to stay in my own inner knowing of what is right for me. You need clear boundaries to enjoy self-love. The only way to do that is to decide what you need for your well-being and say no to all the rest.

As the world changes and enough of us raise our vibration we can lift the planet out of the dangerous place it is presently in, and the key to that is self-love. If we can love ourselves enough to stand up and speak out for our visions of a better future then we can change the planet. It means we stop looking to the externals for love, safety and security. We can choose to walk alongside others whenever we are going in the same direction but we no longer choose to go where they are going *instead* of where we are headed.

So how can we tell if we are moving towards self-love?

We can look at how we spend our time:

- Are we doing something we enjoy for a large portion of our day?

- Are we living with people who bring a smile to our face and our heart when they walk in the door?

- Are we living with people whose eyes light up when they see us?

- Do we smile when we look in the bathroom mirror in the morning?

- Are we making a living that can give us what we desire or need?

- Do we get some time alone for a spiritual practice every day?

- Do we feel connected to Source or God in every moment?

- Do we get some time for physical activity every day?

- Can we take time in nature to restore ourselves regularly?

- Are there voices in our head judging us in harsh ways?

- Have we forgiven our past and all the people in it?

- Do we touch children or animals often?

- Are we creative?

- Are we learning new things that delight and challenge us?

- Do we eat healthy food?

- Do we get enough sleep?

I imagine that list is enough to make you tired. Your own list might be very different but we all know what makes us feel loved and in our right place in the Universe.

Of course, it is easier as you get older and have fewer responsibilities for others. But it is from all of these things, especially the connection to Source, that the fountain of energy you give to others flows. Without enough of this list happening regularly – or any list you might make instead – the flow of outgoing love energy dries up and you start to fall prey to dis-ease in the body, mind and Spirit.

So let's talk about time management as a tool for self-love.

There are the same amount of hours in everyone's day and everyone finds the time to do what they decide they need or want to do. Some people use every minute in a way that will produce benevolent results in their lives. While some people fritter away huge amounts of their time on addictions and time-killers.

What you may have noticed about time is that it is speeding up. Because of the planetary changes occurring; the changing polarity of the sun, increasing sun-spot activity, etc. Time often feels as if we are hitting warp speed. Just yesterday it seems was a fresh new year, now it's May! So I don't want to kill time! I want to embrace time as a friend, extract as much pleasure out of every minute that I can. If I have a job I hate then I change my attitude so that it will go well before attempting it and then get it over as fast as possible.

I threw the TV away 35 years ago and I rarely read newspapers or the media. Our media is completely distorted, and generally run by people who don't have our best interests at heart, so that it is pointless to waste time on it. Almost everything you hear on the news is calculated to fill you with fear and worry. That way you will check in for more. Surprisingly enough, I hear about important events pretty quickly without ever trying.

Let's face it, we can't do much about things happening elsewhere on the planet. We are powerless to change world events. What we can change is our own lives and those of people we interact with. If we do our best to keep our vibration high as we go about our lives then we are making a solid contribution to the world.

How much time do you spend on fun and what actually is fun for you? Being creative is my fun activity and a huge amount of things can fit into that category.

How much time do you spend on exercise and do you enjoy it? Choosing a way to stay fit and flexible and strong that also makes you happy is key here.

How long do you meditate or contact Source in some way every day? On the few days that I don't get this start to the day, my whole day is not quite right. I have a free morning meditation for download that only takes 6 minutes and will start your day off right. Scroll down to the bottom of this page http://healthyover50.com/meditation/

How long do you spend in your car driving during your day? Could you get some inspirational or motivational

103

or educational cds to listen to instead of fussing about the traffic?

Start out with a new mantra. Instead of telling yourself that you don't have time for self-care, say "There is always enough time." Say it often enough that you start to believe it and you will gradually notice your time expanding.

When you are finally done with your daily to-do list you may feel too tired to do any of the mind-expanding things you would like to do. But pick one and do it for five minutes; bounce on the rebounder, do a little yoga, take a little walk, read a new book, write in your journal. Then give yourself permission to veg out after that. You may find yourself pulled into doing something that makes you feel better about yourself than vegging out would.

Family, friends and partners can very quickly pull you away from self-care and self-love. If you have read this book this far you probably give a huge amount of caring to others and they are used to it and will not like to give it up. If they want to watch something totally boring on TV and you usually sit there with them to keep them company, just wean yourself away gradually. Bring a book and earplugs or tell them there is something you have to do. It's important! They can choose to go comatose to life passing but you don't have to.

I bet you can see why I'm a woman who lives alone from that statement ;-)

What I have found to be true with clients and with my own experience is that we all need challenge in our lives, an uphill path to climb. If we take the downhill path of ease and sameness, our whole lives can end up on the downhill run. It is a new challenge that gets us excited, passionate about something, and charged up with positive energy. It doesn't matter what it is that gets you going, it will be different for all of us, just find something and go for it. That's part of my mission now for the rest of my life; to inspire women to jump into life with both feet and do something that only they can do in the world during their second half of life.

Here is the another thought about self-love.

You don't owe anyone anything.

You owe yourself everything! You created your life - and if it doesn't look the way you wanted then you can change it. Don't feel guilty if someone else is affected by your decision to love yourself better. It's an opportunity for them to step up to the plate and love themselves also instead of depending on you. What I have seen is that when we claim the right to self-love fully in our own hearts then other people in our lives start to change in beneficial ways without too much fuss. It is when we are coming from a belief that we don't deserve time for ourselves that others can sense that weakness and pull us back down into service.

Here is a little energetic meditation you can do as often as you need to:

Put your hand on your heart, close your eyes and say,

105

I am totally loved by the Universe - or - I am a beloved child of God.

I commit to loving myself in every choice I make today.

When I master self-love, I will be a force for good in the world.

Thank you, thank you, thank you.

Now, last thing, a mantra I am using right now is, IT'S NOT ABOUT ME!

That may seem to be the opposite of self-love but it's not. I was getting upset about other people in my life who I love who don't make time for me. I was taking it personally. A twist on the old – If you loved me you would.....

Then I realized that most people have more responsibilities than I do right now; they have kids, jobs, partners, passions. They are all running their own dramas and they can't see past them. Unless you are a necessary part of their story you are just more background noise. So get on with your own story and send them love.

We are all so totally supported by the Universe and the Earth and the Elements, and they don't try to make us change our path to suit them like people do. Rest into that for a while. I express gratitude to the Elements on my beach walk every day. Your people will show up again when they are ready to accept you as you are. If they don't then they weren't your people! Don't be afraid of being alone. To love ourselves truly we have to get lots of alone time to explore our changes.

If that sounds narcissistic, it's not. Narcissists need an audience at all times, the more the better. Be joyful for your own full-on attention, appreciate it and it will grow. Presence is the greatest gift you can give anyone, including yourself.

Moving into this chapter:

Be willing to say NO!

You don't owe anyone anything.

Do the meditation.

How do you spend your time?

Kiss the media goodbye.

It's not about ME!

COME HOME TO YOUR BODY

9

SELF-CARING BASICS

I LOVE MY BODY AND FEED IT REAL FOOD

Since I wrote the first edition of this book our food has gone downhill radically. The food conglomerates who make most of the stuff in the markets that they call food, are remorseless in the adulteration of what we eat for their own profit.

From arsenic and antibiotics in cattle feed, to GMO monster foods that are destroying agriculture and small farmers all over the planet, to heartless treatment of animals for food in factory farms and the abuse of antibiotics, it is demoralizing to see how all these things have taken hold of the food chain without raising a stir in the conventional press. Food is cheap and people are happy. But look around you in the market and you will see that something is gravely wrong.

There are many books out now on all these topics so I'm not going to get into it here too deeply, but consider that if you are operating at less than optimal energy levels, if you are developing auto-immune diseases, if you are on multiple drugs for this and that, then perhaps what you put into your mouth is one of the major causes.

Since I am speaking to women over 50, we can all remember when food was actually real; someone grew it or raised it. If we had been offered a 24 ounce cup of soda pop in those days we would not have believed it. Or the ice cream cones that are served up now. Our eyes would have gotten bigger than snowballs. But now greed is the norm and we are heading towards a huge increase in the diabetic and obesity rate over the next 10 years.

So before we can really do the work of being at home in our body we have to feel the full effects of all the gluten, sugar, dairy and other food allergens in our systems. I realize that not everyone is sensitive to these foods – yet – but the numbers are growing every year, and we could all live very comfortable and healthy lives without all of them. No bread, no pasta, no cheese, no ice cream, no sweetened beverages, no artificial sweeteners, no factory farmed chicken tainted with MRSA = a healthier population.

The problem is that even if we made a firm decision to cut out all of the suspect foods, we would run directly into our addictions. The chemists working for the food

110

conglomerates spend all day calculating how much sugar and salt, flour and cheap oils and chemicals toxins they have to add to every non-food to get everyone addicted and reaching for more. It will take an enormous amount of support to get people off of these substances when it is finally proven beyond any doubt how much harm they are doing. Look at how many people are still smoking in spite of incontrovertible evidence that it will shorten their lives. It is really my wish that many of us older women will create the grass roots resistance that turns the tide back to wholesome real food.

Meantime you can read more about real food and the auto-immune diet on my website, http://healthyover50.com/ and that will point you to more sites to learn about the dangers involved in eating our present diets.

So this will be a small chapter just to get the seed planted, if it hasn't been already. As you can probably tell, I get passionate about this topic, partly because I see my grandchildren totally sugar, dairy and gluten addicted and I see how it is affecting their lives. They will not have the capacity for physical or brain health that they could have had, and I'm very sad about that. The world is out of balance when so many children are hungry and so many others are living on chemicalized toxic non-food.

Sleep

Another topic of self-care I will touch lightly on is sleep. There is plenty of research about the majority of people in this culture being sleep-deprived. We would all benefit from 8 hours of sleep every night in a totally dark room.

Here are some tips to get this:

- Wind down your mental activities about an hour before bedtime.

- Get as many hours of sleep as possible before midnight.

- Don't eat for two hours before sleeping.

- Use eye-shades and earplugs to prevent sleep disturbances.

- Leave your cell-phones outside the bedroom.

- If you have a problem on your mind, make peace with it until morning.

The best sleep is deep sleep and we all need at least 30% of it. The primary function of deep, slow-wave sleep may be to allow the brain to recover from its daily activities. It also plays a major role in maintaining your health, stimulating growth and development, repairing muscles and tissues, and boosting your immune system. In order to wake up energized and refreshed, getting quality deep sleep is essential. Without enough hours of restorative sleep, you won't be able to work, learn, create, and communicate at a level even close to your true potential.

I was waking up a lot in the middle of the night, wired and full of ideas, before I started the auto-immune diet. My diet was good but I was still having a lot more fruit than I should. As a type 1 diabetic I really shouldn't be eating any fruit but I love it so I did. Now I've stopped that, plus all

112

the foods that are often hidden sensitivity triggers, I sleep like a log.

I actually bought a fitness tracker that tracks sleep so I can see the areas of deep sleep during the night. It's fascinating! Some nights I get over 50% of deep sleep and I feel so much calmer and more productive during the day. When I was in my high-energy mode, most of my life, I thought people who were calm must not have many creative new ideas to get excited about but it hasn't proven to be true. I have the same amount of ideas but more smooth follow-through. I'm not jumping from one project to another. It's a whole new way of being in the world.

Water

Drink more water. Not the kind in plastic bottles. I got a good whole house filter system and I love water now. A little chia seed or a few lemon verbena leaves in my water makes it even more delicious and healthy. It's all I drink now excepting for water kefir, which is a fermented beverage you can make at home very easily that will repair your digestive system. I was making kombucha for that but water kefir is actually easier and just as good for your system. You can go to youtube to find out how to do it.

I drink a cup of water every time my exercise timer goes off on the hour and do both at the same break, exercise then drink, then back to work. You can't leave drinking up to your thirst mechanism, it has probably been distorted by all the sugar you have consumed over the years.

113

When you pay attention to your fuel of all kinds, food, water, breath, thoughts and emotions then you start to run like a new car, smooth and easy. Once you get into it, you stop cramming fuel into your body that is obviously not going to do it any good. People are so proud of their addictions! It's amazing! They scream at the thought of giving up their coffee, wine, bread, pasta, cheese, etc. etc.

Ok, then – when you do some of the other work in this book and start to really live in your body, then perhaps you will give it a chance to teach you what it wants for fuel.

Moving into this chapter:

Eat healthy, non-processed food.

Sleep 8 hours.

Drink plenty of water, not from plastic bottles.

10

———

KEEP YOUR EMOTIONS MOVING

I TRUST MY BODY TO EXPRESS MY EMOTIONS

Does it feel to you sometimes as if your emotions are like wild dogs that have you by the throat and won't let go; or like germs floating around in your environment looking for a host to feed on? I have some good news and some bad news. The good news is that we are the creators of all of our emotions. The bad news is that we can't *blame* our emotions on anyone else. They are created out of the raw material of our lives and it is only in our resistance to having them move through us that we experience pain.

115

Emotions are energy in motion. They are designed to wash through our body/mind like the waves on the seashore, leaving us clean and new. We can't pick and choose which emotions we are willing to express. When we try to shut out negative feelings, or block their flow through our bodies, all our emotions are affected. The blocks gradually accumulate in our body/mind over the years, leading to stiffness and pain. It is impossible to feel bliss *if* we are unwilling to experience despair. I read recently that testing the immune systems of people before and after experiencing strong emotions revealed that the immune system was strengthened by *both* positive and negative emotions. It is better for us to feel deep grief than to numb out.

Since the second chapter, we have been learning to notice thoughts or habits that we have, or movements that we make. We have been learning to create the witness state. The witness is the part of us that is separate from our behaviors and can merely witness the behavior. You can clearly distinguish by now the witness from the inner critic who watches in order to judge you. The witness is the part that can watch you living your life and be interested and curious about you in a loving, yet impartial way.

The witness belongs to the larger "I" or the Higher Self, who sees *all* of the imaginable possibilities of your life and watches you choose the paths you want to explore. The Higher Self loves you unconditionally and sees clearly how every lesson in every moment of your life leads you on toward home—the alignment of body, mind, and Spirit. The truth is that we are not the movie that is playing out right now in our lives. We are the screen on which the movie plays. We could choose to play another movie any time or we could make a decision that would change our movie forever.

Have you ever dreamed of running away from your life and starting fresh? As a child I longed to run away and join the circus and become a trapeze artist. At other times in my life, I have considered signing up on a sailboat crew going around the world or joining Mother Theresa. Whenever I consider these possible escapes from the movie that I am creating right now, that has become somehow unsatisfying or boring, I feel better about my life. I can more willingly make the small changes I need to make to move on.

So many of us often feel trapped in our lives, but the truth is that we all have choice. There is always a way to run a new movie on your screen if you only want to badly enough. We tend to identify so completely with our roles that we forget sometimes that that is what they are, just roles. It seems to be an ironic twist of fate that natural disasters and wars seem to shake us out of our limited roles and teach us about our resources and capabilities in a way that often surprises us. Crisis often evokes our better selves. We forget our small, daily concerns and rise to the occasion. Within families, long-standing differences and grudges are often given up in the face of severe illness or death.

So what does all this have to do with emotions? I have found that women often have a resistance to believing they can change their emotions at will anytime they want to. Women identify with their emotions in a way that forgets

117

the existence of the witness. You may be playing out sadness or depression in your movie right now but your witness can easily remember a time of peace or joy or excitement or elation.

We have the whole gamut of emotions at our disposal. Our repertoire of emotions as human beings is vast. There is not an emotion that has ever been felt by a human that we don't have access to, and the miraculous thing is, they are all transitory. We can't hang on to any of them without making ourselves sick. Emotions are designed to move through us like clouds on a summer sky and enrich our lives as they pass.

The trick to having your emotions flow through you in a way that energizes your life is to move your body with the feeling. In order to prevent feeling pain, we generally tighten our muscles and restrict our movement. The first thing we do in an uncomfortable situation is hold our breath, and then we tighten our shoulders and our bellies. The fight or flight mechanism is well-known, but the third alternative, to freeze, is actually more common to women than is acknowledged.

Whenever I have been hurt deeply, I freeze into a slightly curled over position, protecting my heart, and I go blank. I couldn't think of a creative solution to my difficulty in this position if you offered me a million dollars. Fortunately I have learned to force myself to move, to get up and walk around, and breathe, so I can come back to life. Coming back to life means that I will have to feel the pain, cry or yell it out of my body, but I have learned that it is worth it to me. My body no longer carries so many of the disappointments and misunderstandings of my life.

The next time you are conscious of deep feeling while alone, notice where in your body this feeling resides. Now breathe into that place and move in whatever way your body wants to. Your body is infinitely wise. It knows what movements will heal you. Freezing, denial, and repression can never heal you. If they could, heaven knows, we would all be healthy. There isn't a woman alive who hasn't tried them all, over and over again.

You may be afraid to try this new behavior. *Do it anyway.*

A voice may tell you that you are stupid or that you can't feel anything in your body. Go inside and watch. Find the part of you that you are holding tight against the flow of emotion. Some part of your body is waiting to move, to squirm, to wriggle, to run away, to scream, or to hit.

We have been taught to repress the healthy expression of our feelings since we were small children. Watch a healthy, small child express disappointment sometime. Her face clouds over, her chin trembles, she starts to cry. If the disappointment is severe enough and she isn't interfered with in some way, she may throw herself on the ground and sob. After a short while, the energy of the emotions will wane and she will get up and get on with her life. Only when children are interfered with, bribed in some way not to feel their feelings, not to move through their pain, will the emotion persist in their body memories or haunt their dreams.

Pain, sadness, and anger that is repressed and not permitted to move through you, will turn into depression. Some of us have had depression of such long standing, like an ever-present blue note running through our lives, that we have completely forgotten what the original pain was about. Psychotherapy works to retrieve the buried memories and we sometimes reach a broad intellectual understanding of the roots of our problems, yet it often doesn't help.

Until we have moved the pain out of our body memory, we don't move on in our lives. I really believe that it is unnecessary to recover the memory of every negative thing that ever happened to us. If your inner wisdom decides you need to remember specific events in order to heal, it will bring them up while you are moving.

If you are moving through your feelings organically, you remember only what you have the inner strength to integrate and deal with. Don't get caught up in the drama of finding out exactly *who* did *what* to you when. It doesn't help you get on with being in the NOW moment in a joyful way You can get trapped in the innocent victim role all over again. Many of us have been playing out that role for *years* already. Let's set the intention to give that one up. When we stop blaming our past, we have to take responsibility for our lives as they are right now, and if we don't like our lives, *we can change.* We are the center of the point of power.

The next time you feel a deep emotion that seems to be recurrent, like always being disappointed when someone doesn't call, even though you know they are forgetful or busy, find yourself a safe place to do some work. Rerun the incident in your mind and notice where you are feeling some sensation in your body.

> Exaggerate whatever sensations you are feeling and put words to them.

> If your throat is tightening, tighten it more, grab it with your hands and say what you are doing to yourself, "I will not let you speak." You are doing it anyway, you may as well verbalize it.

> If your hands tighten into fists, do it more. Say, "I want to hit you!"

> If your feet itch to kick out, do it more.

> If you fold over into a fetal position, do it more. My words for this one are, "I wish I'd never been born." Very dramatic.

That is what we are looking for here—drama---even melodrama. Overact. Be shameless. We are all actors after all. Just keep moving or speaking what you are doing.

If you are numbing out or getting stuck, go back to the provoking incident and re-run it in your imagination. If you are feeling stupid or embarrassed, acknowledge that feeling and keep on acting out anyway. Notice if you remember a time long ago when you felt just the same way. If nothing comes to you, that's fine too. Your intention is to experience the drama so completely that when you are done, it is over with forever.

If you think you are done and then you say something in your head a while later that gets you going again, start over. Notice what you said to bring it back. My words usually were, "It will never be the same." Whenever I am grieving a loss of any kind, I make sure to say those words over and over, and start crying and sobbing all over again, until finally I say it and my whole body responds with, "That's okay. So what. You'll be fine." Then I know I am really done. Of course, if you are grieving the loss of someone dear to you, it may be necessary to repeat this process many times, but each time you will come to a clearer space in your letting go.

When I am dramatizing grief, I will eventually come to a place of peace. When I am exaggerating anger, I usually come to a place of laughter. I hit the pillows or imagine cutting my adversary up into small pieces. If the person is an authority figure, I imagine them in ridiculous situations. I get very creative with my vengeance until finally I laugh until my ribs hurt. Don't feel guilty about wishing your adversary harm. We are not so powerful that we can hurt people with our thoughts in such a short space of time. Harboring long-standing resentment hurts the people in our lives much more.

This process of clean anger usually leads me to deep forgiveness of my adversary's actions, and my own, and I can see us both more clearly and gain insight that will head off future misunderstandings. Most people out there in the world who make us angry are just triggering our childhood pain anyway. That is why I try not to confront anyone when I am upset. I own my feelings and work on them by myself first; then I am clearer about what needs to be said to resolve the situation without blame.

Blaming someone else may be ego gratifying in the short term, but it never works to make me feel better in the long run. When I have resolved an upset in this organic way, I feel bigger, my heart feels open and warm, I feel good all over. When I am still in the grip of blame and justification and control, I can often win because I am clever with words, but my heart is still small and it still hurts. Do you know that feeling? To me it says I'm not done yet, there is still more work to do.

If you go through the whole process and come to a clear space and the person you are upset with is still back at the level of the upset, that's okay. We can do our work, but we can't do theirs for them. Give them some space and love and they will either come around or they won't. It isn't important any more. The child in us often fears that our anger or sorrow is bottomless and endless, but when we do this moving process we always come to the bottom if we act out enough.

We may fear that our anger will lead us to kill someone, but anger stored up in our body cells will more likely end up killing us. By working alone on our anger, we can take responsibility without hurting anyone else. In the clearing out of every deep emotion in this way, as we feel it, we have the ability to heal our past while we deal creatively with our present.

Timing your Emotions

It seems as if it is rare in our busy lives to be free to deal with our emotions as they come up. Something may

123

trigger old pain or an over-reaction in the middle of our workday or in a place where we are expected to act professionally. To be true to our feelings in the moment is a wonderful way to live, but it is idealistic. In the real world, we often have to put our emotions on hold until a more appropriate time. I believe that as long as you promise yourself to deal with the emotion later, and keep your promise, you will not lock the blocked emotion in your body tissue.

For example, if you become upset at something that happens during a business meeting, you have three choices. You can protect yourself so completely that you don't even hear it. I did that for years. When I was home alone I often realized that I was sad and forlorn, and I would have to re-run my day to discover the reason.

The second choice is confrontation. You can hash out the disagreement right there and then. Most of us have so much old baggage of hurts and upsets that can be triggered innocently by the behavior of a colleague that this is a risky choice. When you are upset, you are revealing much more about yourself than you realize.

The third choice is to hear the words, witness and acknowledge your reaction, and immediately promise yourself to work on it later alone, and then get back to the business at hand. Upset of any kind will trigger our child personas within, and the last thing most women want to do is to relate to colleagues and bosses with all the tender feelings of a four-year-old.

If you think you can't put your feelings on hold in this way, try to remember a time when you were forced to do so. In emergency situations, I have often been the person who handles the crisis perfectly, only to collapse later. We do have choice. Have you ever been sad over a loss, maybe a death, when the whole world looks gray to you, and someone takes you to a funny movie? You find yourself laughing and forgetting your pain. When you walk out of the theater it settles back on your shoulders.

When my father died, I had to continue working although I wanted to just curl up in a ball somewhere. I assumed my professional persona and put my grief aside for my working hours. I would have all the emotions normal to my working environment. When I left work something would remind me that my father was dead. The old "nothing will be the same" voice would start up and instantly I would become dispirited and gloomy again.

Try to remember a time when you were feeling exceptionally happy and lighthearted, and you were with a friend who had suffered a loss. You put your gaiety on hold and became sympathetic and caring. We have all done it. In childhood, we were usually discouraged from feeling our feelings in the moment, so some psycho-therapeutic models of the past thirty years have presented the opposite. Let it all hang out whenever. Now we can let the pendulum center back into the middle and express our feelings when it is safe in the moment and save them for later when it's not.

This week, practice putting your less intense feelings on hold to experience later, A minor aggravation or irritation, a small sadness, would be a good starting point.

125

Notice if you are consciously acting, holding the thought of your original emotion under the pretense of another. That isn't what I mean. See if you can actually step into another role in your repertoire that doesn't even remember the negative emotion.

Think of it this way. The actors in a soap opera are very unconvincing to me. They seem like people who can't forget for a minute that they are acting. A really good actress, Meryl Streep, for example, makes me forget for two hours that I am watching actors. What is going on in the movie seems real.

A friend of mine was giving a party and her husband said something to her in front of their friends that she thought demeaning. She pretended to have a good time until the party was over and then gave him a piece of her mind. She had allowed a careless remark to spoil her evening. I'm sure that has happened to all of us. If she had been able to move completely back into her party hostess role and enjoy herself, without rerunning the remark and nursing the hurt feelings underneath, she could have had a good time. Then when she brought it up later, it probably could have been clarified quite quickly. Her husband loves her dearly and had just been momentarily unconscious. It happens to the best of us, especially in party situations.

Often, when we nurse our hurt feelings in this way, it is for a purpose. We have the mistaken idea that we can change other people if only they see how much they have hurt us. Or we have the fear that if we don't show them our pain, they will do the same thing again, or worse. We are hanging on to our negative emotions in order to manipulate others. It doesn't work. So many of our behaviors don't work, and yet we refuse to give them up.

My first marriage was my schoolroom in this regard. I tried to manipulate that man to get my needs met every way I could think of for seventeen years. It never worked and I have to tell you I was infinitely creative. I finally had an Aha! experience when I realized that he was doing what was right for him and I had to do what was right for me. I made up my mind to always remember that I can't change anyone but me. So there was no longer any need to hang on to my pain to influence others. I can just go ahead and work on it myself and get over it sooner and get back to feeling good. That was a relief!

Moving into this chapter:

Here are some of our choices around emotions:

- We can choose what we are feeling.

- We can choose to put our feelings on hold until we are safe.

- We can choose to work old pain out of our bodies by using all the incidents in our daily life that trigger the past pain for us.

- We can choose to use our body sensations to work through pain.

- We can stop deadening ourselves by repressing our feelings, and own them instead.

- We can stop using our feelings to manipulate others.

- We can explore the wonderful sensations that come from the free expression of joy and grief and all the other unlimited emotions that enrich our lives.

- We can acknowledge that we create all of our feelings, good and bad. No one does it to us.

11

ARE YOU AN EMPATH?

I AM ONLY RESPONSIBLE FOR MY OWN EMOTIONS

I didn't really get it that I am an empath until about ten years ago. I always felt different and I knew that I could read other people's emotions clearly, but I didn't realize that more than half the emotions I was feeling were not my own. When this light dawned on me my life became much easier.

We are all empaths to some extent, it's part of the feminine psyche, but some of us have the talent to an extra and uncomfortable degree. I used to wonder how my mother knew when I did something I shouldn't. Now, when my grandchildren try to fool me, I can see all the cues

129

she was picking up from body language. But empathy is a big part of that knowing also.

One clue to your amount of empathy is the depth of your emotions as a child. Was everything either agony or ecstasy for you? It was for me. I cried buckets as a child. When I read a book like Jane Eyre in class, I would cry all night for all the orphans and all the injustice in the world. My mother had no clue how to comfort me and lost patience, so I learned to cover up my emotions as best I could.

There are energetic and emotional components to empathy. So the next time you suddenly feel sad and really can't think why, ask yourself what just happened. Did you read something about someone in trouble, did you pass by someone who was obviously in pain, or did something big happen in the world, like an earthquake or a rebellion?

Before I acknowledged my empathy, when I became inexplicably sad, I could always rattle through my brain and find some good reason very quickly. I could launch into an old story or an old movie and justify my sorrow in a heartbeat. But that led to regurgitating my stuff and didn't ever lead me to more light.

Now when I feel myself experiencing emotions that don't feel congruent with my present moment, I ask myself, "Who does this belong to?"

If my body says right away, "Not me!" Then I can send the emotion back to whoever it belongs to, or I can send it down to the earth for recycling or up to Source to be transformed by light.

It's a simple process. First center in your heart, put your hand there if you want to, and visualize the emotion in your body. How big is it, how heavy is it? Then imagine it soften like coconut oil in the sun and start to flow. It can flow down to the earth, up to Heaven or out through your heart, whichever feels best. Keep on encouraging it to flow until it is all gone. Then you could say, " I open to all emotions beneficial to me in this moment and I allow all others to pass me by. Thank you angels," (or whoever you usually thank).

Right now on Earth (2014), we are going through huge changes. We are moving out of 3 dimensional living, moving higher. The Earth herself is being transformed in huge ways, from solar flares, asteroid activity, whatever. There are many reasons why things are changing so radically here but no-one can doubt it is happening. Tsunamis, earthquakes, weather changes, government and economic changes – we are in a tornado of change. This can be very uncomfortable and bring up a lot of fear. If you are an empath you can take this fear in and think it is all yours.

It's not! Trust me! 85% is from other people. You just have to have enough fear inside you to resonate with it and that will attract it to you.

So one solution is to try to stay away from negative people. Don't hang out with them. If you are a sensitive, an empath, you can't afford to spend a lot of time with people who have habitually dark, fearful or angry energies.

Another important thing is to ignore and tune out the media. The media is a tool of fear and gives a totally distorted view of reality. The media manipulates people's minds. They want you to be fearful because then you are controllable. Even some of the alternative media sites online have been infiltrated by the manipulators. Be careful what you read or listen to. Consider all fear based information to be noise and energy pollution.

Most people are very resistant to giving up their media. They say I'm a Pollyanna and I won't know what is going on in the world. Well, it's funny, without seeking out information, I always know when major world events happen. I just don't know all the details of all the ongoing strife in the world and I don't care to. I gave up media 35 years ago and I'm sure that's why I get more done that most people. I'm not distracted by things I can't help or change.

For empaths it is essential to realize and acknowledge what you can help with and what is none of your business. Even when we see family members in pain or emotional distress, it is usually none of our business. If we help others do things they should be figuring out for themselves, we are actually cutting them off at the knees. When we aren't there with the helping hand, what will they do?

All women have the helper gene, but particularly empathic women spend enormous amounts of their energy helping others. Partly because that makes life easier for them! If everyone in the world was happy right now I would be totally blissed. But I'm not responsible for making everyone else happy. That's an inside job. We all came in to our human bodies to learn our own lessons and I have to say that my hardest lessons have taught me the most. I wouldn't be the person I know and love if my life had been smooth sailing from the getgo.

Tuning out the world

For some parts of my life, especially when I got sick in my fifties, I became a kind of hermit. I tuned out the world and concentrated totally on getting better. My family is small and lives far away so I was on my own. I did have the computer! So the computer became my helper substitute. It was a good substitute actually, because I wasn't compelled to take it's advice so as not to hurt it's feelings. I could try stuff and discard it if it wasn't for me.

But I went through many dark nights of the soul during that long time and I came through it changed. My optimism and openness to the world had taken a hit. I always had a deep connection to Nature and the Elements but I no longer felt very connected to the world of humans. I feel compelled to say right now that I'm sharing this because I know it has happened to others. When we go through a lot of darkness alone we can get stuck in tuning out the world. It wasn't there for us when we needed it, so forget it!

But tuning out, becoming numb, or shielding is never the answer. Because you can't just shield yourself from the darkness, you are also closing to the light. I gradually realized this as I came back to health and I am once more open to the world and to humans in general. We are all in this together and we have to stop abusing this planet before it gives up on us. We have to drop our defenses and open to

133

all the light we can hold so we can move forward as far as possible.

I see the answer as being open as much as we can in our daily lives. When I move through dark energies, coming up in myself or coming from others, I center back into my heart, take the hit and transform it into light and then move on. I don't take it personally, I don't add another layer of blame and shame. It's like when my puppy has diarrhea and I find poop on the floor. I just clean it up and move on.

I hope some of this helps a bit and I want to say a special thank you to all the empaths who have incarnated right now to help the world at this crucial time.

Huge blessings to you!

Moving into this chapter:

Ask if the emotion you are feeling is yours. If not, send it back to whoever it belongs to.

Clearing emotion:

First center in your heart, put your hand there if you want to, and visualize the emotion in your body. How big is it, how heavy is it? Then see it leaving your body, moving forward, down or up, whichever feels right in the moment. Then, when it is gone, you could say, " I open to all emotions beneficial to me in this moment and I allow all others to pass me by. Thank you angels (or whoever you thank)."

Get free of media. Most of it is detrimental to your peace of mind. Some of it is an attempt at mind control.

12

—

LET'S GET PHYSICAL

MY BODY GIVES ME PLEASURE

When I ask my clients what it is that brings them pleasure in their bodies, I have become used to their startled reaction. Pain they know all about. Pleasure they're not sure of. They think for a while and then smile and say, "Sex!" as if that must be the answer I am looking for. I remind them of the pleasure of having their skin stroked, by a partner or by soft clothing, or the pleasure of lying in the sun in a garden on a spring day. "Yes, of course," they say, "I had forgotten that."

They have forgotten because they aren't usually present within their skin to experience any sensation. To be truly present with our bodies is to be ready and willing to experience totally, with all of our senses, and without comparisons. It is a left-brain tendency to pull ourselves out of an experience in order to compare it with another one. To our sensation-seeking right brain, there never was another experience just like this one and never will be. This is complete and this is enough.

When were you last fully present to feel some of the following experiences:

- A long, hot, sweet-smelling bath or shower.
- Massaging your body with lotion or oil.
- The sun shining on your bare skin.
- A warm wind or rain touching your skin.
- The smell of flowers or wood smoke or new-mown grass.
- The sounds of music.
- The warmth of a wood fire, crackling, dancing, and glowing.
- The sensual pleasure of tasting a wonderful meal.
- The freedom of walking under the stars on a warm night.
- Moving through water.
- Dancing in a freeform way.
- Laughing joyfully with your whole body.
- Singing.
- Stretching languorously.
- Making love.
- Yelling.
- Sucking something, our first pleasure.
- Running.

137

- Exercising.
- Moving in a full range of motion.
- Spinning like a child until you lose your balance.
- Skipping and jumping.
- Climbing a tree and sitting in it.
- Walking out in nature after a rain.
- Planting things in a garden.
- Stroking someone.
- Cuddling with someone you love.
- Touching an object that was made with love.
- Bringing yourself to orgasm.
- Smiling with your whole body.
- Hugging a friend.
- Petting an animal.
- Playing with a child.
- Hugging a tree.
- Lying on the grass watching clouds pass by.
- Watching the waves move in and out at the beach.

What did I leave out? What are your own special pleasures?

This week will be an adventure into the seeking out of our pleasures. We will find whatever gives us the sensation of total delight and completeness. When we are in a state of sensory pleasure it feels as if we would be content to continue forever, and yet gradually, in our own time, we become complete with it, and move on to something else with no sense of loss.

Notice your reaction to becoming more aware of pleasure.

Are you impatient? Who has time for that kind of thing?

Do you feel guilty? Does the voice of duty say you are supposed to work, or bring pleasure to others, but not to yourself?

Does your pleasure consist solely of getting out of your body—reading, watching television, eating addictively? Even listening to music can be an out-of-body experience if you have to sit still in a hard chair and restrict your aliveness in order to hear it, I can't listen to music any more without moving. I used to sit in a row at the symphony listening with my ears and my mind, but now I need to listen with my whole body. Thank goodness for electronics!

What does the word *sensual* mean to you? It is very different from sexual, isn't it? Picture in your imagination a woman dancing alone in a sunny meadow or a cat stretching on a windowsill. Cats are so perfectly present in their bodies in every moment. Just watching a cat stretch and roll and play makes me want to get down on the floor and join in.

Many of us lost touch with sensuality at an early age. It is a quality that has long been regarded as dangerous, even sinful. Taking pleasure in our own senses, especially touch, has been looked on with disapproval, especially for women. This is a country founded on puritanical roots. Let's free ourselves of those old restrictions and move joyfully into the realm of the senses.

Explore each of your senses in a way that makes you feel completely present in your body. Using your soft gaze, look at someone or something you love as if you were caressing them. Looking at a person in this way is like discovering them all over again. Allow your eyes to wander over a beautiful plant or a hand-crafted object. Then look at yourself this way in the mirror, as if you had been blind to your own beauty, as most of us are, and just regained your sight.

If you want to try something really extraordinary, blindfold yourself for half an hour and wander through your house or garden, noticing how your other senses become more alive. When you take off the blindfold you will see the beauty around you with new eyes. Just looking at the way the sun beams in the window, casting shadows on the walls, can fill you with a sense of the beauty and wonder of life.

Now try sound. Listen to music with your whole body Do nothing else. Just feel the music flow through every cell in your body. Don't resist, don't block.

Now get lost in your sense of smell. Fill the house with incense or cinnamon or perfume or flowers. I have planted my garden full of fragrant flowers, and whenever I can, I bring in enough to make the whole house smell. Jasmine by the side of my bed has woken me up in the middle of the night with its intensity. I lie there and float in the smell and it drifts through my dreams. No wonder perfume was considered an aphrodisiac. Right now the mimosa trees are in bloom and I have branches from them in every room.

Dedicate an entire evening to taste. Taste all the different flavors you have in the house as if experiencing each one for the first time. Let different tastes melt on your tongue—a kiwi, vanilla, honey, vinegar, some salt.

The last is my favorite, the sense of touch. Touch everything that gives you pleasure. Touch objects with your eyes shut and sense what you can from connecting surface to surface. We can survive the loss of all of our other senses, but not the sense of touch. Without sufficient touching, babies will die or fail to grow. How many of us actually get all the touching and stroking we need to feed us emotionally? Touch can heal so many of our ills. It is far better than any medicine.

Touch your face as if you were learning to recognize it in the dark. With gentle hands, feel every part of it, every nook and cranny. Do you think you could recognize your loved ones by touch alone? Get out a sweet-smelling lotion and stroke it into your skin, or take a hot bath and brush your body gently from head to toe as if you were preparing yourself for an initiation.

Dancing

Dancing is such a natural, wonderful expression of sensual joy in the moment. Joyful children dance and sing without inhibition. Then a time comes when self-consciousness sets in. We start to look at ourselves from the outside and we lose our spontaneity. As we grow up, our dancing becomes choreographed and formal, and it becomes important to do it right. Then we train our bodies to move only in the ways that are acceptable to our peers in the style of the moment. Let's forget all that and remember how to move freely for the pure joy of it.

Since many of us are threatened by the whole idea of dancing, even alone in our own space, we will start with something wonderful and easy. First, erase all images of *Dancing with the Stars* from your mind. We are going to redefine the word dance as any movement that gives us pleasure. That eliminates success and failure. Anyone can apply. No previous training required!

Be alone in a room with some free floor space and play some music you love. Play it *really loud.* This is important. Use headphones if you have to, but it is so much better without them. Lie on the floor in a comfortable position with your arms on the floor beside you and allow the vibration of the music to flow through you. It is an incredible experience. The drums will be playing one part of you, the flutes another. Soon your every cell will feel as if it is dancing. The music will be playing *you.*

Experiment until you find the right music. Classical music with full orchestra is perfect. Vangelis is great. Try *Heaven and Hell* or *Chariots of Fire.* If you have The *Planets* by Hoist, play Mars when you are tired or depressed and Venus when you are wired. Ballets are better than opera for this. Music can change any mood in a moment. Great music affects us deeply on a cellular level. You are probably aware that different kinds of music have different effects, so for this experiment, allow your cells to choose for you.

The second time you experiment with this exercise, allow the music to move you in very small ways. Let your

142

muscles contract and relax to the music wherever you feel it in your body. You may find you have muscles you were never aware of before. The music can persuade tight muscles to let go. Gradually move more and more until you are actually rolling around on the floor like a happy baby—stretching, reaching, rolling, curling, and stroking. Move in circles. See if you can make every joint in your body move in a circle. Circular movements are so healing to the body.

Touch yourself as you move. Some of us never touch ourselves at all except in the shower. Bring your hands alive with sensing and curiosity, and stroke yourself as you roll around. Doesn't your skin feel good? That is real sensuality—the good feelings your senses bring you. Smell your own special smell. Taste yourself. Have you ever noticed how children suck their arms and their knees as well as their fingers and thumbs. When your inner critic tells you to get up off the floor and stop acting like an idiot, tell it to get lost until you are finished. This is your time to play.

We are creatures. We have bodies. Our minds and our intellects would have us forget that, but our senses long for us to remember it.

Our bodies can be the chief source of comfort in our lives. No one else knows us like our bodies. No one else is always there for us, no matter how much they love us. People leave, people die. Take your pleasure and your comfort from your own body. Don't worry if it isn't the size or shape you would like. The pleasures of the senses are not limited to a certain weight or appearance, thank goodness. If you allow your body to please you, and live inside it more, it will adjust to its own healthy shape.

There was a time when I resented the way my skin was changing as I got older, and then I had a wonderful experience in the shower one day. I was feeling low-energy and disconnected. I looked down at my arm and suddenly I really saw myself. Isn't it amazing how you can have a shower every day for months without really seeing yourself? I saw my skin, the microscopic creases in it that lead from one tiny hair to another. The way it sparkled with the water droplets in thousands of rainbows.

My mind can always find a problem to brood over if I allow it. It is endlessly inventive. But my body and my senses are always there in the moment, available to be tuned into and to bring me back to the magnificent present.

Sexuality

Sex in this culture is often such a commodity. Sexuality is a hard subject to approach. For most of my clients with severe pain, it turned out that their sexual experiences in the past or present were an important component of that pain. Women throughout the ages have endured so much emotional and physical pain in order to gratify their own and others' sexual urges. We have to recognize that we carry the resonance of our heritage from centuries of abuse and bondage.

We also feel, on some deep level, all of the abuse being inflicted on women right now, all over the world. We can deny this connection all we want. We can feel safe within our own relationships, but the fact is that women are not yet safe on this planet. In most places, we cannot walk alone at night. We are often not safe in our own homes. This is the undercurrent that stirs deep and dark beneath all our fears of our honest expression of our sexuality.

When women talk together openly, it seems that every woman is willing to admit to some difficulties with her own sexuality. Either we have no partner, or we have the wrong partner, or we have the right partner but the wrong technique, or we have no time, or no privacy or we are too stressed out. The list goes on.

During our lifetimes, there has been such change in the traditional roles in this area of life. Yet healthy sexuality can be a way of expressing every changing face of union, from an ecstatically spiritual blending with the divine to a deep exploration of our creaturehood.

Sexual energy is one of the most powerful, universal energies we deal with in our lifetime. Keeping it repressed costs us more than we realize. We use up so much energy in burying our sexual feelings that we cause our bodies to stiffen up and start dying. My intuition is that in order to start to heal ourselves and others, we have to honor our own sexuality first.

Some of us were taught as young girls to cut off both sensuality and sexuality until Prince Charming arrived and then everything would be splendid. It wasn't. Then came the sexual revolution and women were acknowledged to have sexual needs equal to men—equal rights to orgasm. For many women that didn't work either.

Most women have needs for emotional bonding and a sense of security before their sexuality can be fully expressed with another person. We have to reclaim our own sexual bodies and learn to pleasure ourselves first. When we can explore and delight in our sexuality alone, to the point of orgasm, then we can be truly safe. Orgasm is good for our bodies. It enhances the immune system. If we can give ourselves that gift joyfully, we can move into choice in the area of relationship.

Many women I know have made the choice to live without a partner of either sex. They feel the need to pursue their spiritual path through life basically alone, with the love and support of their friends. This is a perfectly valid choice and certainly a common one throughout history. It is also a fact that women live longer than men and many women are alone through no choice of their own. Whether or not we choose the path of relationship is not the issue. The issue is that if we hold the key to our own sexuality, then we can keep ourselves healthy in the moment by giving *ourselves* the gift of orgasm.

The way we have most effectively controlled our sexuality is by holding the pelvis rigid. By doing this, we create an energy blockage in the whole area of the genitals and lower back so that we will not have to feel the feelings that arise there. Any time we hold any part of our body rigid we are affecting our whole lives. Rigidity spreads.

146

If I hold my pelvis stiff, I cannot walk freely because my hips can't rotate, and then my arms don't swing loosely so my shoulders get tight. Lower back pain is often related to a chronically tight pelvic area. Hip and knee problems develop from the same cause. If you don't give a hoot about orgasm, never had it, never want it, then do this exercise for the health of the rest of your body.

You can watch this video at
http://comehome2yourbody.com/videos/

- Lie on your back with your knees up, feet on the floor.

- Repeat each movement at least ten times, slowly, gently, and lovingly. Be fully present.

- Imagine the clock face on your body as you did in the rocking breath. Twelve is at your heart, six at your knees, three is at your left hip and nine at your right hip. The center of the clock is your tailbone touching the floor.

- Start rocking your pelvis slowly from twelve to six and back. This is a small, soft movement. Your bottom does not pick up off the floor.

- Now rock from three to nine and back. Don't flop your knees from side to side. The movement is in your pelvis.

- Now go around the clock in a circle from twelve to three to six to nine to twelve. Make your circle as round as possible. If you go slowly enough, you will notice the places where your circle is not round.

147

- Reverse the circle. Remember to move gently and
  sensually.

Gradually, as you practice this movement every day, you can add more numbers to your clock and fine tune your awareness of where your pelvis is in the circle. The muscles that move the pelvis are among the strongest in the body and freeing them up to move will affect every movement you make. You can also practice these pelvic circles while sitting and standing. When done standing, they are reminiscent of belly dancing or the Hawaiian hula.

After you practice pelvic circles every day for a while, you will probably notice that you are feeling more sensual. You may start to be more aware of your genital area. You may feel the flow of energy from your sexual center for the first time. Many of my clients were afraid of this feeling. They were afraid they would be compelled to do something they would be ashamed of, like going to a bar and picking up a stranger.

Getting in touch with our own flow of sexuality doesn't make us suddenly out of control. Opening up to the experience of our feelings doesn't mean we need to express those feelings inappropriately We can always learn to bring ourselves to orgasm with a little experimenting and practice.

Be gentle with yourself. Seek out the pleasure centers of your own body. Men have limited their erogenous zones to a small area, but for women, our whole body can be an erogenous zone. There are sex manuals for women to learn from, but if you give yourself the freedom to explore, you probably won't need them. Make up a fantasy in your imagination. You are unlimited. You can create anything that pleases you.

Women often turn to vibrators to pleasure themselves, but I have found them to be too mechanistic and lead to multiple, shallow sensations rather than a full orgasmic release. Many times women have told me that they need a male to come to orgasm because they like the feeling of penetration. I thought so too until I learned the next exercise. No video on this one since it is mostly internal.

Lie down with your knees up the same as before, and experiment with contracting all of the muscles of the pelvic floor. You will be tightening everything as if you needed to go to the bathroom and you couldn't find one. Contract and relax at least twenty times.

Next, try to isolate the muscles of your vagina from those in your buttocks. You will probably not succeed completely at first. Do the best you can. A way to practice this is to start and stop the flow of urine next time you go to the bathroom.

When you have the control of the muscles in the vagina isolated, think of the opening of the vagina as the first floor in a seven-story building and gradually tighten up on each floor as you climb up to the top. Some deep, internal belly muscles will be activated. Tighten gradually and relax gradually—up and down as if you were riding an escalator in the building. Make sure the muscles in your buttocks are as relaxed as possible.

This exercise approximates the feelings of penetration and has enormous benefits. It will encourage orgasm if you are pleasuring yourself. It will make you a more exciting lover if you have a partner. It will help you to avoid the problems of collapsing organs later in life, and it will aid in preventing you from having problems with incontinence.

The whole media marketing program pushing diapers for women makes me angry. This is not a natural part of aging. Don't buy into it. Lack of movement and lack of stimulation for the muscles of the pelvic floor lead to incontinence, and both can be corrected. We can make internal changes in our muscle tone instead of relying on external props. I taught a friend of mine to do these exercises in one session and she called later and said she had been practicing in the car and had spontaneous orgasms all the way home.

If you are embarrassed to even think of experimenting with your own sexuality, ask the shy teenager or the disapproving parent within you to wait outside the door for a while and just try it. All of this is normal behavior for adult women and is nothing to be ashamed of. It is your body. Learn to enjoy it completely while alone and you may choose to share that pleasure with a partner at some point in time when you are ready. If you have a partner, don't feel guilty for experimenting alone. You aren't being disloyal. You are learning something that will ultimately benefit you both.

Isn't it funny that you couldn't say the word "menopause" in polite company twenty years ago and now we never stop hearing about it. Many of my postmenopausal clients who are alone put sex out of their minds and bodies with relief, leaving "all that" behind them. If this applies to you, you may not have even read parts of this chapter, thinking you don't need it.

Turning off our sexuality is not good for the body The hormonal system is one of our "use it or lose it" systems, and the hormones we manufacture when we are feeling sexual benefit our bodies in many ways. Osteoporosis is endemic in this culture among older women, and the activity of our hormonal system vitally affects the health of our bones.

It is sometimes difficult to begin your sexual life anew when you have given it up so completely. Start out by allowing yourself some sensual experiences, memories, and thoughts. Stop censoring yourself. Find some fiction of the exact kind of sexuality that stirs you, or make up your own fantasies.

When I have been busy on a creative project for a while, it sometimes occurs to me that I haven't felt sexual for ages. I think my intuition reminds me. So I give myself a sensual evening, a date with myself—music, bubble bath, everything to set the mood. A part of me seems to sigh and say, "Thank goodness. I thought you had forgotten me."

I will finish this chapter with a Feldenkrais story. In my training we loved these stories. My master teacher was giving a demonstration of Feldenkrais work in front of a group of doctors. The client was an elderly woman who was in extreme pain with her back and very stiff all over. He started to work with her, gently moving her as far as her restrictions would allow. As he got closer to her pelvic area, she stiffened up even more and started to clench her fists. Finally, as he rocked her pelvis gently she started pounding the table and yelling, "No!" She was as surprised as he at this reaction.

What came to her awareness was that she was terribly angry with her husband, who had died six months before. They had enjoyed loving sexual relations right up until his death and she had tried to deny her loss by stiffening up entirely. After the session her pain was gone and she was able to move through her anger and grief and get on with her life.

*This week, choose your own homework from all the material in the chapter. Ease in slowly, be kind to yourself, love yourself, and keep a sense of fun.

13

GETTING IN THE FLOW OF ENERGY

MY ENERGY FLOWS CLEARLY FROM MY HEART

Like all living things, we are all unique patterns of energy that have danced their way into matter. We float in an endless field of energy that most of us cannot see with our outer eyes. We have luminous, bright-colored clouds of energy all around us, and our energy fields embrace each other long before our bodies ever connect. Science is finally measuring and photographing these fields so that they can be proven to the entire satisfaction of the left brain. Our right brains see, feel and know information intuitively, without words, and our left brains mock anything that cannot be explained and measured. This split is healed only when we invent better tools to measure what cannot be seen. It has happened throughout history. People in the West, who honor the left brain above everything, didn't believe the world was round until they proved it, didn't believe in germs, didn't believe in flying.

Now there is a new paradigm shift occurring. The old Newtonian world view has changed to the new view of the Quantum universe. The Newtonian way of looking at things was simple. It was a mechanistic world view. We are all separate and when we do things to each other we set up a chain of reactions, like billiard balls colliding.

The new ideas of Quantum Physics say the same as mystics have claimed since recorded time began. We are all one. I don't have to collide with you to affect your life. I can affect you merely by being in your energy field, or even by living my own life in my own way. The Chaos theory says that a butterfly fluttering in China can create a pattern that may become an electrical storm in New England. We are discovering anew, on the leading edge of thought, how connected we all are. The flow of energy is the magical medium of connection.

Remember a situation you were observing, not participating in. You could have been at an airport or in a crowded room and someone you could see was behaving in a way that either touched your heart or made you angry. Without any personal involvement, you have been affected. Are you separate from that event now that it has touched you?

When I think of images that have touched millions of people deeply and initiated great change, there are two that come instantly to mind. The picture of the little Vietnamese girl running with her clothes burned off from napalm was seared into my memory and was a crucial turning point in public opinion about the Vietnam war. The first pictures of the Earth sent back from outer space changed forever the way many people connected with their planet. In the same way, a movie or play or novel can deeply affect the way we see our world. Remember a movie you saw recently that changed the way you thought or felt about some issue.

Now remember an occasion when you saw a person for the first time and felt immediate attraction or repulsion. What were you responding to? Was it body language? Was it their resemblance to someone in your memory banks? Or was it the subtle energy field, called the aura, that emanates from all of us? We all read these fields unconsciously as we go through our day, but some people read them more clearly and are less easily fooled than others. You *can* learn to read these energy fields consciously.

Think of an adjective to describe *yourself* as you meet someone for the first time. How would a person who never saw you before describe you in one word—shy, arrogant, controlling, beautiful, kind, overbearing, depressed? Would they see the real you in that description or are you projecting a convincing image? Most of us would like to give the impression that we have our act together, that we have all our ducks in a row.

My brother, Derek, calls some people he meets Posers, meaning they aren't real; they are hiding behind an act. Are you a Poser or do you allow who you are and what you are feeling in the moment to show? Do you think you can detect a Poser? When you improve on your natural ability to read the energy fields of others, they will not be able to fool you. You will know when someone is angry, and whether that anger is their habitual state or just a fleeting emotion. You will know when someone is feeling truly happy and powerful, or just covering up inner sadness or fear with a cheerful facade.

Whenever we are false, other people know it on some level of awareness, if not consciously. Remember a time when you were with someone who was putting on an act. We can either play along with the act ourselves or we can cut right through it by being clear and honest. It seems to me that there is a lot less pretense now than when I was a child. It was always very confusing to me when grown-ups said one thing and I could clearly see that they were feeling the opposite.

Do you remember the honesty and clarity you had as a child? Can you imagine a world in which no one could lie and get away with it? It is my belief that we already live in that world but, as in the story of the Emperor's New Clothes, no one wants to be the first to acknowledge it. Our energy fields always reveal exactly who we are and how we are feeling, they give us away.

Our energy field extends out around us and becomes subtler and subtler, like mist. Close to the body, it has various colors that indicate our state of mind. Inside the

157

body, which is the denser part of our beingness, the energy runs most powerfully on certain meridians or pathways. Different ancient philosophies, such as the Indian or the Chinese, have slightly different patterns of pathways. The spinal pathway has seven chakras or energy wheels at seven locations on our spine where certain different energies are expressed.

If this is all new to you, it may well sound like New Age baloney. It is actually very ancient wisdom, so bear with me. When you experience the energy running through you, you will know the truth of it. Until then it is just words.

If you have been doing the Heaven and Earth breath regularly, by now you have probably experienced the sensation of energy in your heart or moving up your spine or through your hands. People experience this sensation in various ways—as heat, light, tingling, or shaking.

When I send intense energy while doing healing work, my hands actually vibrate. Some of my clients have thought I was nervous or tired because they don't feel the flow of energy, just the shaking. Do you recall the image of heat on a road stretching into the distance on a hot day, the mirage effect? That is how it seems to me. A shimmer that can get more and more intense, leading my hands into a kind of trembling.

Experience your Heart Energy

Sit quietly, cross-legged or on a chair with both feet on the ground. Close your eyes and imagine a wheel spinning at the level of your heart between your breasts. This is the heart chakra. It is the center of love energy and is the easiest to access at first. Bring into your mind an image of a time when you deeply loved someone or something innocent, like a child or a kitten or a flower. Feel the energy of that pure, simple feeling intensify in your heart like sunshine. Know that this feeling of love is all around us all the time, waiting for us to open our hearts to receive it.

With your imagination, turn up the volume on that feeling until you feel a physical sensation in your heart, a stirring. You may feel your heart brimming over, as if it holds enough love for the whole Universe.

It is often necessary to keep the mind focused on a simple task so it quiets down and gives you some space to experience. If your mind is busy with thoughts, concentrate on repeating the words, "I am love." Imagine that the words come out of your heart. Breathe deeply, exhale fully.

When you feel a clear energy in your heart, send it down both of your arms to your hands just by willing it to flow there. You may feel them tingle or light up in some way. Now put your hands facing each other about a foot apart and create a bridge across the space with the energy you are sending. You can feel the energy jump across the space to connect and form a circle from your heart through your hands and back again to your heart. Relax your shoulders. You don't have to force anything, just surrender and allow the energy to move through you.

When you are finished, pull the energy back from your hands to your heart, take a couple of deep breaths, and let it go. Does it feel as if you reached into a bottomless well of heart energy? Do you feel revitalized and optimistic?

Pure heart energy, the energy of unconditional love, is the primary energy of life. We send out many energies during the day, the energy of our emotions, anger or fear, perhaps, but when we can tune into the heart center and send out love, then we hold the key to healing both ourselves and others. I think the awareness of energy traveling through the body and between people is finally beginning to come into the mainstream. When enough people feel it and accept it as reality, critical mass will suddenly be reached, and then most people will be able to feel it without special preparation.

Consider all energy explorations a game. This is not drop-dead serious. Too much effort makes it harder to learn. Take it lightly. Many people think that if they imagine something, it is not real. The fact is that everything we create is created first in the imagination and then in reality. By opening to the possibility of feeling our energy moving through us, we eventually enable ourselves to actually feel it. Sometimes we have to tune in to that particular channel on our receivers for a while before the message comes through.

It is much easier to learn to move energy from a person who does it well and can induct you with their presence, but with patience and trust you can also learn alone. Don't allow yourself to feel like a failure over this. Thinking that you can't do it is the fastest way to block energy flow. Given time and intention, anyone can experience energy.

People have difficulty feeling something as obvious as their own pulse at first. Think of how many substances are flowing around and through our bodies all the time outside of our conscious awareness—blood, lymph, cerebrospinal fluid, hormones, etc. Is it so hard to believe that energy does the same thing? It is like our own personal electrical system. It can't be seen directly, but it's effects can surely be felt with a little practice. When I work with groups of beginners and they start to feel the flow, there is always such a sense of joy, even relief. People realize they have been missing an important element of their lives.

Feeling our energy consciously is a quantum leap on the road to home. Home is the place where we remember we are immortal, boundless, limitless, and living from a sense of peace and wonder. We are all so much bigger than our day-to-day struggles, but we get caught up in our dramas and forget. Practice this exercise of sitting and growing your awareness of pure heart energy as often as you can.

This universal love energy that connects all things is not a personal love, it is an unconditional love, and it is our birthright. A few people throughout the ages have always been able to feel it. They are the ones we have called mystics. Now the ability is spreading so that we can all have access to this unconditional love state whenever we choose.

Within the Christian tradition, Jesus worked extensively with energy. He said, "Anything that I can do, you can also do and greater." The laying-on of hands that Jesus did was simply the transmission of healing energy. Many nuns and nurses are using the same techniques today. Therapeutic touch is one of the names given to this kind of healing.

Frequent practice really helps. Many people would like to learn to see auras and seem to expect to see clear rainbows of color with their physical eyes. I have found that feeling energy through the heart center is the best and safest road for most of us. There is less danger of being caught in ego power states. Seeing auras is much easier, if you want to, after you have felt heart energy run through your own body.

The most widely accepted energy system is the Spinal Pathway with the seven spinning chakras. It is an ancient system from the Vedic texts of India.

There are many books available that deal more completely with the various chakra systems. My intention is to give you enough of a structure so that you can more easily experience the energy for yourself.

The first chakra is the root chakra at the base of the spine and connects us to the earth, to the physical plane and to our physical life, health, work, finances, etc. Do you know someone who has this energy in abundance? They will seem very grounded, very down-to-earth, very practical. The color is red. When you do the Heaven and Earth breath, this chakra is awakened by the earth energy you pull

162

up your spine. This chakra is involved whenever we have issues with our security. People who are unawakened in this chakra are likely to be very spacey and unrealistic; they don't seem at all sure that they want to be here on the Earth in a body.

The second chakra is the sacral chakra just above your pubic bone and is the sexual and creative chakra. Think of someone you know who is sensual, not overtly sexy since that is often an act, but someone who enjoys the whole world of touch. This color is orange.

You will feel this chakra ignite when you are attracted to someone sexually. Have you ever been having an ordinary conversation with someone and suddenly a sexual spark lights up between you from a look, a touch, a certain word? That is your second chakra reminding you that you are a sexual being. You don't have to act on it, just enjoy the reminder. Since this chakra covers the whole world of creativity as well as sexual creativity, you may find during periods when you are without a love partner that you are suddenly creative in many other ways.

The third chakra is the solar plexus chakra above your navel and is the emotional chakra as well as the power center. Do you know anyone who can express her feelings honestly in the moment and then move right back to peace and joy? This color is yellow. This chakra is highly volatile and its desires also don't have to be acted upon. Just notice which emotion is being played out and appreciate it. A person who has a lot of energy centered on their emotional chakra often tends to be involved in power struggles.

163

This is also the energy center of the body, called Chi in the Chinese system. It pulls in energy from the sun even when you can't see it in the sky.

The fourth chakra is the heart chakra, the love center. This color is green. This is the center for all kinds of love, including the highest—unconditional love.

Few people can manifest this kind of love that sees all and expects and needs nothing in return. It is the love our Higher Self has for us. This chakra is the center of our energy system and is the most in need of awakening right now. Whenever you are in doubt about anything in your life, bring your awareness back to the heart center and rest there. This is where the energy of the earth and the energy of Spirit are equally at home and can mix to bring balance to our lives.

The next chakra point, located between the heart and the throat, has no number because it is not mentioned in the old systems. Brugh Joy calls it the high heart chakra. It is an energy point that has to do with regeneration and rejuvenation. We are developing and changing as spiritual beings all the time, as we are evolving, and it is very important to open to and appreciate this chakra.

The fifth chakra, at the throat, is the energy of true and wise speech and of verbal creativity. Think of someone you know who always says the magical words that heal your heart. This color is blue. If your sexual or emotional chakras are over-active, you can set the intention to balance the energy up to this chakra and you will have a burst of creativity of some kind.

164

The sixth chakra is at the third eye between the eyebrows and has two energies, that of the mind and that of the inner wisdom. Do you know anyone who lets their intuition guide their life, listening to the voice of inner wisdom on all decisions? Your mind can very easily lead you astray since it is often run by the ego, but your Inner Wisdom never will. This color is indigo. I usually finish my meditation by connecting the energy of my heart center with this chakra, seeking to see clearly from my heart and my intuition.

The seventh chakra is at the crown of the head and is the energy of Spirit. This is where we connect with Source and Home, our limitless self. This color is clear bright light or in some systems, purple.

The ideal is to have the energy running through all the chakras in a perfect balance for you on your particular life path. For instance, at some points in our lives, and even some points in our monthly cycles, the energy in the sexual center will be more pronounced, other times less so. We usually feel more energy at the emotional center when we have internal upset and disturbance in our lives and the root chakra activates when external change and turmoil come into our lives.

The important thing is to appreciate the flow of energy, not allowing it to get stuck at any one spot. We will know when we are blocked because, like a stuck record, we will keep repeating the same thoughts over and over, thoughts of need or lack or problems. Our bodies will also reveal energy blocks by becoming stiff or unresponsive or painful. At those moments, breathe deeply or dance or do

165

the Heaven and Earth breath to get the energy flowing again.

We do not actually create energy ourselves, although it often seems as if we do. We merely channel the energy from the sun or energy that is all around us all the time. Like electricity, no one knows exactly how it works. We take in pure energy from the field around us and by tuning into our thoughts and feelings it can come out through us as love, fear, anger, despair, hope, joy, or a million other patterns. It is the same energy. What we create with it is our choice. Just as we can choose to use the breath and the food that we take into our bodies for playing or working or fighting or resting.

It may sometimes seem easier to create anger or drama in order to get a stuck situation moving again, but we could just as easily choose love. By resting into our heart center and repeating "I am love" for as long as it takes for our energy to shift, we can choose from a position of feminine power.

No matter how stuck we are, we can always ask our Inner Wisdom for help in seeing the larger perspective or the perspective of the heart. We have only to be willing to give up our ego needs to be right or to be in control. That's all! No big deal!

Every time we interact with someone else we are exchanging energy. If you remember that your energy field extends out from your body, it is easy to understand why you are more comfortable with some people close to you than others. The distance our field extends around us varies according to how open and expanded we feel. Sometimes when we don't feel safe, our aura becomes dense and is very close to our body. When someone approaches, we can tell in a millisecond whether this person is safe and what energy they are sending us. So much of our communication goes on energetically before we ever *say* anything.

Spend a few days noticing the quality of your energy and how you send energy to others. Check which way the energy is flowing between you. Are you expanding or contracting, giving or receiving? Do you feel fed by your interactions? Think of energy as the invisible component of support or encouragement. Who is doing the feeding, the supporting?

Now for more practice. From a distance, watch pairs of people interacting and guess who is sending the most energy and who is receiving or resisting. When you are learning by watching others, some clues for the direction and quality of the energy are body language, facial expression, and voice animation. It is interesting to guess which quality of energy people are sending. From the mind chakra, the energy can be in the form of stimulating conversation or debate, the exchange of ideas. Even listening to someone's ideas with interest is sending energy from the sixth chakra. From the fourth chakra, the energy is always love. From the emotional chakra, we can send energy in the form of any emotion we choose. Sometimes the energy will feed people and sometimes it will deplete them.

For example, if you are being pathetic, you are unconsciously asking for a dose of energy. If your friend is a

167

nurturer, she will provide the supportive energy for you. If your friend is not inclined to give you the energy of support, she may get irritated at your neediness and send you the energy of anger. You have still been fed with energy and you may still feel more alive than you did before. This is how children learn to attract negative attention and feed from it.

There are very few interactions in which we send and receive equally. Notice if you are always sending energy, pouring love and help into your friends' empty spaces. Many friendships are unequal in this way. In a healthy relationship we take turns, sometimes giving and sometimes receiving.

Also notice when you overwhelm others with your energy They will often physically step back. Love or anger can be overwhelming to many people and much of the energy we send out has demands and needs attached to it.

Very few people are sending out unconditional love energy in their lives. We take the basic, unconditional love energy of the Universe and we move it through our chakra system and transform it into something less pure. In the same way, electricity can light up a concert hall or activate the electric chair. By becoming clearer and more honest to ourselves and owning our emotions, we become clearer transformers of this universal energy.

Notice also that most people have set limits on what they can give or receive. Feel your own limits. Are they different with different people in your life? Energy is the same as any other gift that someone can give us. From some people we can accept a present and from some we cannot. We can also tell instantly if a gift has strings attached. What we do most of the time is to establish boundaries around ourselves so that we can feel safe. Imagine these boundaries as wooden fences.

Notice how high your fences are with certain people, and how they vary with your mood. When your fences are high and dense, notice the reaction of people around you. Watch other people's fences fluctuate. When you notice that someone's fences are up, send them a gentle blessing of pure love energy or give them an encouraging word or a touch and watch the fences disintegrate. It is a true test of the level of heart energy we send out to another when their defenses crumble and they feel safe in being vulnerable with us.

Notice also if you are willing to be vulnerable to others. We are all so afraid to risk. We censor so much. We often hold back on our vibrant aliveness, the intensity of love and joy we have access to feeling and sharing. This is a choice we make moment by moment to fit in with the people around us.

I remember in my family if I was happy or exuberant, my older sister would manage to punish me somehow. But if I was depressed or upset, I got a payoff of attention from my mother. So guess what I learned! I have a firm belief that our natural state is joy, and like bubbles rising in boiling water, it will emerge any time it is able to. At eighteen, I traveled six thousand miles to be alone in a new country so I could find my way back to joy. There is a driving force within all of us to be whole and to experience our feelings and our energy fields freely.

When you begin to become aware of your interactions with others on an energetic level, you may notice that you feel drained and depleted after being with certain people. We all have our own store of personal energy that we create by breathing, moving, and eating. You can imagine how much this store can vary according to the depth of our breath, our eating habits, and how much moving around we do. Even if you are very active and eat wisely, your personal store of energy is finite. By tuning into the universal supply and becoming a channel of energy as you learned in the Heaven and Earth breath, you can tap into an unlimited source of energy that you can draw on at will.

There may be times when you feel unable to draw on this universal source because of the negativity of the situation you are in at the moment. To avoid becoming depleted by the negative energy of others, you can easily learn to protect and shield yourself. Here is a tool you should practice alone before you need it so that when the time comes it can be used almost instantaneously.

Imagine yourself surrounded by a diamond of clear light. This is the light of Spirit. This diamond of light can protect your energy field from intrusion and keep you from harm.

Energetic Touch

When you touch others, always be aware of how powerful touch can be. Touching someone with energy running through your hands, and with your heart open, is a gift we can give anyone, anywhere, anytime. In the medical system in this country, there is not enough credit given to the healing power of touch. If you touch someone as you would a loved child, they will feel better. If you touch someone without loving awareness in your hands, you can take care of their bodily needs, but they will feel isolated and invaded, like an object.

It is an inspiration to me that so many nurses are learning the various techniques of healing touch. I was in a spiritual group with many women who are nurses and they are tired of being medical technicians. They know the power of touch, energy, and words on sick people and they wish they had more time for that kind of personal involvement.

I recently asked my Inner Wisdom how people could get sick at all when we are always surrounded by healing energy. I wanted to know the purpose of a healer. The answer I got was that a healer is someone who can focus the energy and direct it. Electricity needs wires and plugs, radio waves need receivers, laser beams need some kind of focusing machine. Healing energy needs us.

Science acknowledges that electricity, radio waves, and light are around us all the time, but without focus they are not useful. We can all learn to focus healing energy. It is not difficult at all; but don't confuse healing with curing.

171

Don't always expect your energy to make a person well. There is too much we do not yet know about why people get the illnesses they get. Sometimes the energy we send to someone who is very sick will help them to move through the dying process more easily. Let them be the judge of what they do with your gift.

At a time when your heart is closed and you have a lot on your mind, touch someone you love and notice their response. Another time, with the energy of love flowing in your heart and in your hands, touch them again in the same place without saying anything, and notice the different response. If they are caught up in their mind and closing out feeling, they may not react in an obviously different way immediately, but usually, being touched with love will bring anyone back into their body

I'm a California hugger. A hug is a very good test of the ability to send and receive energy. You can hug ten different people and you will have ten different experiences according to how much energy they are willing to let flow between you. Have you ever hugged someone and felt as if they weren't there?

It is such a blessing when family members are in the habit of hugging hello and good-bye. Both people can tell immediately, without words, how the other person is feeling. Whole body contact reveals so much. The energy exchange is so direct.

I believe the only useful way to communicate deeply on matters of importance is heart to heart with energies open and flowing. Anything less will result in some level of misunderstanding. Since we all come from our own experience and our own family background, we just *think* we are speaking the same language. It is an illusion. Everyone has a different intonation of meaning for the words, the tone of voice, the intensity, and the context. It is actually a miracle that we can communicate at all. It is only because we are picking up clues from our intuition and energy fields that we understand as well as we do.

Notice how clear you can be when you are fully present, speaking from your heart to someone who is willing to be present in listening. Most of the women in the groups I have been in agree that to have someone listen to them with complete attention and acceptance is the most healing thing in the world. We don't need most of the advice we are given; we just need to be heard.

Energy is such a fascinating subject for me. I just love it, and this is merely a beginning of the exploration. I hope you have experienced enough of the actual flow of energy to acknowledge its reality. By keeping this awareness in the back of your mind, you will learn how to relate better to your own energy patterns and cycles, as well as to others.

Remember that we are never the same. In every moment we have a different expression of our energy field. We are constantly changing like a beautiful kaleidoscope. Wanting the safety of the known, we try to stop our own flow through our lives, and that is where we block our natural spontaneity and joy. Let yourself flow, with the ups and downs, the rhythms, the cycles, the seasons, the tides of your emotions, your needs and desires.

173

Feldenkrais said it is desire that drives us through our lives. Our needs are basic to all of us—food, shelter, clothing, etc. Our desires are unique to each one of us, and it is the drive to satisfy these desires that causes us to move and expand and grow. Without desire we would be like stagnant ponds. Desire pulls energy in from the Universe for creation. That is the pattern of a fulfilled life, curiosity and desire pulling in healing, love, and wisdom energy for creativity and expansion. If we settle for anything less than that we are selling ourselves short.

Moving into this chapter:

Practice the sitting exercise as often as possible, pulling energy into your heart.

Study energy flows between people.

Watch interactions from a distance and practice reading which way energy is flowing.

Imagine the seven chakras in your own body. Before you go to sleep at night, put your hand gently on each location and send energy from your heart to open each chakra. Ask your Inner Wisdom to balance your energies while you sleep.

Experience the different energies you can send out from the different chakras. Send a friend sexual energy, joy, anger, love, and wisdom, and ask them to guess which you are sending.

Practice sending energy from your heart to light up your hands, and then touch children or animals or someone who is sick.

174

14

CONNECTING WITH SPIRIT

I NOW ALLOW SPIRIT TO GUIDE ME
EFFORTLESSLY THROUGH MY LIFE

I cannot imagine moving through my days without access to my Inner Wisdom, my Higher Self, and Spirit. Without them I would feel small and lost.

I will try to define what these terms mean to me in *this* moment, at this stage of my life.

Inner Wisdom refers to the small voice within that tells me when I am centered and on track in my life and when I am not. It is the little sense of discomfort I get when I am about to make a mistake. It is the desire that prods me to go somewhere or do something that turns out later to be a necessary step on my path. My ego and personality levels want what they want, and they want it NOW. Without my Inner Wisdom to balance me, I would go rushing off in pursuit of pleasure only to find that it doesn't truly satisfy me. My Inner Wisdom has access to information from other levels of reality. It is responsible for my flashes of insight and intuition.

My Higher Self is a personal guide. She speaks only with the voice of deep wisdom and never leads me astray. She loves me completely and unconditionally. She is the larger space within me that sees my life unfolding and knows I am on my path toward fulfilling my mission in life as best I can. She also knows that whatever emotion I feel in this particular moment will pass, and that is a truth my ego often forgets. In many religions it is said that we are all gods and goddesses. My Higher Self is the part of me that is closest to realizing that goal.

Spirit is the connection with the larger Universe of which I am a necessary and unique part. I am a drop of water and Spirit is the ocean, limitless and boundless. It is from the place of Spirit that I can heal and see other people clearly, and it is my connection with Spirit that gives me the strength to let go of something I love when I need to.

Visualization

I am going to start with a visualization exercise designed to help you meet your Higher Self if you haven't already.

I will record an mp3 for you with this visualization that you can download from my website here - http://comehome2yourbody.com/audios/.

People have often told me that they are not good at visualization or imagining things. It turns out that they expect to get a clear image on the inside of the eyelids as if they were running a video inside their head. No one I know sees images in quite that way. Think of a purple elephant. Most people do not get a clear picture, but see it more like a dream, where trying to hold on makes it slip away. It is as if the file in our brain for purple and the file for elephant are both activated at the same time but the resulting image doesn't go through our visual apparatus.

Think of a lemon. Think of a hug. Now close your eyes and imagine a house burning down. Was it a big house? Was it a Victorian? Probably yours was not, but mine was. You are looking with your inner eyes. Change your expectations of visualization from an eyelid video to a dreamlike awareness and your contentment with the process will improve enormously.

Lie down on the floor or sit very comfortably and close your eyes. Breathe deeply into your belly and relax every part of your body, starting with your toes and working up to your forehead. Take all the time you need.

You are walking alone in a grassy meadow in the spring sunshine. There are flowers everywhere and the birds are singing all around. You can smell the grasses and flowers as you walk and a feeling of complete peace and well-being comes over you. You feel at one with the Universe and you raise your arms to the sky and give thanks for the beauty of the day.

You keep walking and catch sight of a beautiful building in the distance. You immediately know that it is a sacred temple and you are irresistibly drawn toward it. As you walk closer, you realize that there is a deep ravine between the meadow and the building, and you stand at the top not knowing how to cross.

You look toward the left and notice some rough steps cut into a path leading down to the bottom of the ravine and you know that they were carved by women like yourself who have been here before you. You count the steps as you go down, deeper and deeper. It gets darker as you go deeper out of the sunlight, but you feel something pulling you forward, and finally you reach the bottom.

At the bottom of the steps there is a stream and you wade across in the shallow water. When you get close to the other side, you see a deeper pool and a sparkle in the sunshine catches your eye.. You slip out of your clothes and plunge into the warm pool. You pick up a beautiful, shining crystal from the depths and hold it to your heart.

On a rock beside the first step leading up to the temple there is a special robe waiting just for you, and you put it on and start the upward climb. Every step brings you closer to the top and you have a deep inner knowing that someone is waiting for you there who has loved you always. Finally you are at the top and you walk forward to the entrance. You stop for a moment on the threshold to center yourself, holding the crystal at your heart, and then you move into the dim room lit with shafts of sunlight from the high arched windows. The light falls softly onto an altar and you move toward it.

On the altar is a large crystal bowl full of water, and a voice within you says, "Look within to find the one you seek." You eagerly look into the water and see your own face reflected there, and for a moment you are disappointed. But as you look deeper into the eyes looking back at you from the water; you see a wisdom and an inner beauty that you didn't know you had. You gaze deeper and deeper and the image changes slowly until the face looking back at you is infinitely wise and infinitely loving, and your own voice says, "Welcome home."

The voice asks you if you have a question to ask of your Higher Self. You speak of what has been most on your mind and wait for the answer to come back to you. You treasure this wisdom from the deeper part of yourself and ask how you can meet her again when you need her. She says that she is always there for you and will come and speak with you whenever you open to her: You decide on a signal that will show you are ready to listen to your deepest wisdom.

The time has come for you to leave so, with your heart full of appreciation, you place upon the altar the crystal that you found in the pool. You move back out into the sunlight feeling new and vibrantly alive, happy as a child to have seen the one who has walked beside you for so long. You retrace your path down to the stream and change back into your own clothes. Then you cross the stream and with a light heart you climb up the steps into the bird songs and flowers of the meadow.

The music of nature gradually fades away and you return to the awareness of your body in this room, keeping the lightness and joy and the sense of homecoming with you as you open your eyes.

If you are in doubt at any future time whether the voice inside you is the voice of your Inner Wisdom or the voice of your ego, you can signal your Higher Self in the way you chose at the temple, and she will tell you. Any small ritual will call up her presence. You could sit in the lotus position for an hour or you could jump in the air while clapping your hands. She doesn't care what you do. She is always there for you and will answer any call. I used to ignore what my Higher Self said if it didn't fit what I wanted to hear, but I have learned over time that she sees a larger picture of my beingness than I do. Now I trust her completely.

It is one of the major benefits of being born into a female body that women can connect directly with Spirit. It is part of our genetic heritage. There are many differences between men and women in the physiology and chemical makeup of the brain. The part of our brain that enables the right and left hemispheres to communicate is the corpus callosum. This part of the brain is forty percent larger in women than in men, and this difference enables women to balance the logical, rational mode of the left brain with the spatial, intuitive mode of the right brain.

In my opinion, it is because many men have difficulty in connecting with Spirit directly that most religions in the world are set up and controlled by men. They have the dogma, we have direct experience. Women don't need a cathedral, a prescribed ritual, a designated intermediary, or a long list of rules. What works for each of us will be different according to our life pattern and preferences. Whatever gives you bliss in your life will bring you Home.

One quick and easy way for me to access Spirit is the Heaven and Earth breath. I do it at the beginning of meditation. Then I clearly state what I want to be and do in my life at this time and my willingness to do the work involved, then I thank my angels and guides and allow appreciation to flood through me, and I just sit. I watch my breath to keep my mind quiet. Sometimes I get blissed out and sometimes I get bored.

Spirit in Nature

Being in nature is one of my most well-worn paths to bliss. If I am off-center or upset, I go for a walk on the beach or sit with my back against a tree. I have a deep need for that kind of contact and I get crabby without it. I have to go to the redwood forest for a few days every once in a while to get back my perspective on this crazy world. I put my whole body up against the thick bark of a thousand-year-old tree and I feel in my cells how nature endures and prevails.

I have a favorite eucalyptus tree beside the ocean near my house and if I'm tired or upset, I go there and sit up amongst the sweet smelling branches gathering solace from the sounds and the smells of Earth.

Nature makes me feel humble, and yet not insignificant, as if I am part of a huge plan and my small part is vitally needed. I feel more willing to do my part just as every tree and blade of grass does theirs. I have always lived close to an ocean. The pulsation of the waves is completely healing for me. All of nature has such ebbs and flows, the constant changing of the light and the seasons. That helps, me to appreciate my own highs and lows, my fluctuating, warm and cold currents.

Art and Beauty

Art and beauty are also clear voices of the Spirit. There is special beauty in an object that is made with love. It speaks directly to your heart. Once I was in a large city in Switzerland, and I was feeling lost and scared. I was fighting with my husband and the fight felt terminal. Walking through those cold, dreary, gray streets in the middle of winter, without one leafy tree to bring me Home, I was in despair. We went into a cathedral that had some famous stained-glass windows and suddenly my breath was taken away by their beauty. I sat and let the colors rain down on me and heal my heart. It was magical. I was touched by the Divine. When I walked out of there our argument melted away under the light of pure love.

Creating anything with love is a gift to the world. We all have the power to create beauty A wonderful meal, a poem, a drawing; we can all start somewhere. Try any art or craft that attracts you and be generous with your praise and appreciation for your efforts. Center in your heart and let

183

your Higher Self work through you. That is how I have always done all my artwork of various kinds. Sitting down at the potters wheel was like entering sacred space for me. My Higher Self is so infinitely creative.

Music and Dance

I have never been able to play a musical instrument, but for many people music is a true path to Spirit. Even listening to certain music moves your energy into higher chakras. Pachelbel's Canon never fails to transport me to another realm. Chanting is also something that can take us very deep, and anyone can do it. It works especially well in a group. Drumming is also getting to be a popular way in our culture to access altered states.

And, of course, music brings us into movement, ecstatic movement. Most primitive cultures use dance or movement of some kind to bring them to an experience of the Divine. In our own country the Shakers did the same. What wonderful lives they had, such peace and simplicity and order, and then releasing into spiritual ecstasy by moving.

There are many places now where you can do different kinds of freeform movement, just listening to the music and letting your body move in the way it wants to. Search for Soul dance, Journey dance, Ecstatic dance, 5 rhythms and many more and you might find a group nearby. Group energy magnifies the effect of our intentions geometrically not arithmetically so that makes it extremely powerful.

It is only on writing this chapter that I realize how many ways I have to make my connection with the larger Universe. When I am healing with energy I step deeply into Spirit. No matter how I feel before a session, I am also healed by the end of it. Any form of giving can have that effect for me. Giving anything from the heart can bring us Home.

A woman in my spiritual group said that certain scents connected her with Spirit. We all collected herbs and sweet-smelling flowers from the garden for someone who was going to court for a legal battle. We imbued the little bundle with our loving energy so that she could hold it in her hand and smell it and remember that she was not alone.

Gratitude

When we let go of our daily dramas and step into gratitude for all the good in our lives then the doors of our heart fly open. We can feel the golden light of Spirit flowing out into our world. Right now, write down 5 things you are grateful for and 5 people too. See if that makes you smile. Then write 5 things about yourself you are grateful for. When I do that I always resolve to spend more time in gratitude because it makes me happy. Dwelling on what needs some work or isn't quite perfect does not get me to the same space.

Ritual

It is no accident that all ancient and primitive cultures, without exception, devised rituals to contact the Divine. It is a great loss to women that our rituals have been forgotten. Think how valuable it would be to have some open acknowledgment of a relationship's end. If a loved one dies, we have a right to mourn. If a lover leaves us or we leave them, we feel as much pain but we have no receptacle for our grief. We have no ashes to scatter and no body to bury. Even normal, healthy losses, like a child going off to college, are unmarked.

A ritual is the process of marking an event that is significant to us. It is a marker stone on our journey through life. Moments of joy and moments of sorrow should be marked amongst us, and the presence of Spirit could be invoked for comfort.

Think of the rituals you have in your family. Are they the same as you had as a child? Most of our rituals are around celebration times—weddings, births, holidays. Have, you made up any rituals for your children or grandchildren on the spur of the moment? Children love rituals. They demand repetition. You just have to do something twice with a child and they say, "We *have* to do it. We *always* do that."

Nowadays we have allowed gift giving and food sharing to take over as our ritual, to say what we cannot say in words. A few years ago, I started creating rituals, making them up as I went along. We made up a ritual for the daughter of a friend on her first menstruation and a wonderful blessing circle for a new baby. For the baby we offered a gift from our hearts, a quality we wished for her to express in her life. The variety was creative and surprising.

I perform a ritual on the new moon to thank the moon that has passed and to bless the month to come. I pull in all the energies for everything I want to create in this moon cycle. I bless the new plants I put in my garden and invoke the flower spirits to care for them. Little things, but they enrich my life. Ritual used to be a private thing for me. So many people are embarrassed by it. It feels strange and weird at first. Now it is becoming popular and I am often asked to lead a ritual or a blessing or a ceremony. It doesn't matter what you call it. You are invoking Spirit to commemorate an event in your life and Spirit is always blissfully happy to respond.

I was in a spiritual group of women who met regularly. We did guided visualizations, healing with energy, working with dreams, writing, rituals for various occasions, and book discussions. We could always think of something to do that made us leave lighter and clearer than we arrived. We didn't plan far ahead so that we could be free to explore the mood of the group.

We opened with a deeper version of the Heaven and Earth breath and then shared how our lives had been since we last met. We laughed a lot. Mostly we supported each other in bringing Spirit into our daily lives. The group was really working for us. I moved away and then I got sick so I haven't had a group since then.

The power of Spirit is magnified by joining together. Try it. Begin by mentioning to women you know that you would like to start such a group. There were fifteen of us at our first meeting and some decided that it wasn't what they wanted. We ended up with usually about ten and that seems like a good number.

It turns out that writing and now revising this book has become a deep, spiritual experience for me. I made a ritual ceremony, set the intention to help women, called in a blessing, and gave the book and the revision up to Spirit. It is amazing how it progressed after that.

It certainly is true that it is by teaching that you learn. For years, when women asked me why I wasn't teaching, I would say I wasn't ready yet. That's so left-brained. We are all teachers for each other and, with the guidance of Spirit, we can spread compassion, love, and laughter in our lives.

Moving into this chapter:

Remember a time in your childhood when you felt connected to Spirit.

Remember a loss you suffered that was never acknowledged, and create a ritual to honor that loss. You can use incense, candles, flowers, water, fire. You can have a burial in the earth of your hopes and dreams. You could draw or write something and burn it. Let the part of you that knows how to do ritual take over.

Be in nature daily and connect with Spirit.

Connect with someone you love from the level of Spirit and see them absolutely clearly. Let go of everything except appreciation.

Get in touch with the way you contact Spirit the best, your own special way. Clarify it to yourself and ritualize it so that it will be available to you even when you are in distress.

CONGRATULATIONS

You have finished the book. If you were doing a read-through, then it's time to love yourself enough to start again and really do the work.

If you've done the work, you are one in a thousand! I know you have already made huge progress in coming home to your body. Enjoy your new life!

My wish for you is joy, love, peace, comfort in your body, mind, and Spirit, and a deep connection with your Inner Wisdom and Higher Self.

Blessings!

I would very much appreciate a review on Amazon if you found this book helpful. There are so many books being published now and they are found by the amount of reviews they get, so if the readers don't speak up and add their opinion the books don't get seen. You can also sign up for the newsletter on the http://healthyover50.com site and get many new tips and videos on having increased joy and health in your life. I have a couple of new book ideas mulling in the brain cells now that I have the basics addressed in this one, so you'll be the first to hear on the newsletter. One will be on a new version of a meditation labyrinth that I have created which is specifically suitable for these changing, hectic times.

ABOUT THE AUTHOR

P am Free has studied movement since her training as a Feldenkrais Practitioner in 1989 and she practiced energy work before that. She is passionate about teaching women to reclaim their power and connection to Spirit through movement and awareness; the everyday movements of everyday lives. She has also studied many different alternative healing modalities, working on cleansing childhood issues and misunderstandings out of the body, so that women can be their best selves in the NOW moment and not be run by old programming.

Pam went through a mysterious severe illness in her 50s after she moved into a home that was harboring hidden mold. It took many years to recover using her own research on the internet to discover and try healing tools of all kinds. She has many tools she has developed that were proven through that time of self-study and self-healing, so the book has been completely revised and new chapters have been added so you can have the latest information to cope with the changes coming into the world of women.

In the hermiting stage of her illness Pam was able to connect deeply with her guides, both external and internal, and she is being told now to move forward and bring her own particular wisdom into the world. We all have something to share that could benefit others and now is the time for us to move forward and be seen so that we can join together with others of like mind to shift the vibration of the planet.

Now Pam is loving life on the California coast, creating her new website of tools for women, from the mainstream to the woo-woo, at http://healthyover50.com She is writing, teaching, coaching, dancing, learning the trapeze and embracing all the amazing new energies pouring into the planet in these tumultuous times.

COME HOME TO YOUR BODY

www.ingramcontent.com/pod-product-compliance
Lightning Source LLC
Chambersburg PA
CBHW060252290526
45789CB00001B/305